THE ARCHITECTURE AND DESIGN OF MAN AND WOMAN

ALSO BY ALEXANDER TSIARAS

FROM CONCEPTION TO BIRTH

ALEXANDER TSIARAS

TEXT BY BARRY WERTH

THE **MARVEL** OF THE **HUMAN BODY**,
REVEALED

THE ARCHITECTURE
AND DESIGN
OF MAN AND WOMAN

DOUBLEDAY

NEW YORK LONDON TORONTO SYDNEY AUCKLAND

PUBLISHED BY DOUBLEDAY
a division of Random House, Inc.

DOUBLEDAY and the portrayal of an anchor with a dolphin
are registered trademarks of Random House, Inc.

Book design by Eric Baker Design Associates, Cindy Goldstein

Library of Congress Cataloging-in-Publication Data
Tsiaras, Alexander.
   The Architecture and design of Man and Woman:
   the marvel of the human body, revealed/
   Alexander Tsiaras; text by Barry Werth.
   p.cm.

   ISBN 0-385-50929-4
   1. Human anatomy—Atlases. I. Werth, Barry. II. Title.
   QM25.T48 2003

Printed in the USA

November 2004

FIRST EDITION

1 2 3 4 5 6 7 8 9 10

I WOULD LIKE TO THANK:

ATTILA AMBRUS FOR HIS LEADERSHIP, ENDLESS CREATIVE ENERGY, AND EXTRAORDINARY TECHNICAL AND AESTHETIC SKILLS.

JEREMY MACK FOR HIS ATTENTION TO DETAIL, HIS VISUALIZATION SKILLS, AND TREMENDOUS TALENT.

AND TO THE ENTIRE TEAM: LASZLO BALOGH, ANN CANAPARY, MARK MALLARI, KARINA METCALF, JEAN-CLAUDE MICHEL, BETTY LEE, MATT WIMSATT, AND POY YEE, WHOSE COLLECTIVE ENERGY, INDIVIDUALITY, CREATIVE INSIGHTS, AND LONG HOURS HAVE CONTRIBUTED TO A NEW LEVEL IN SCIENTIFIC VISUALIZATION.

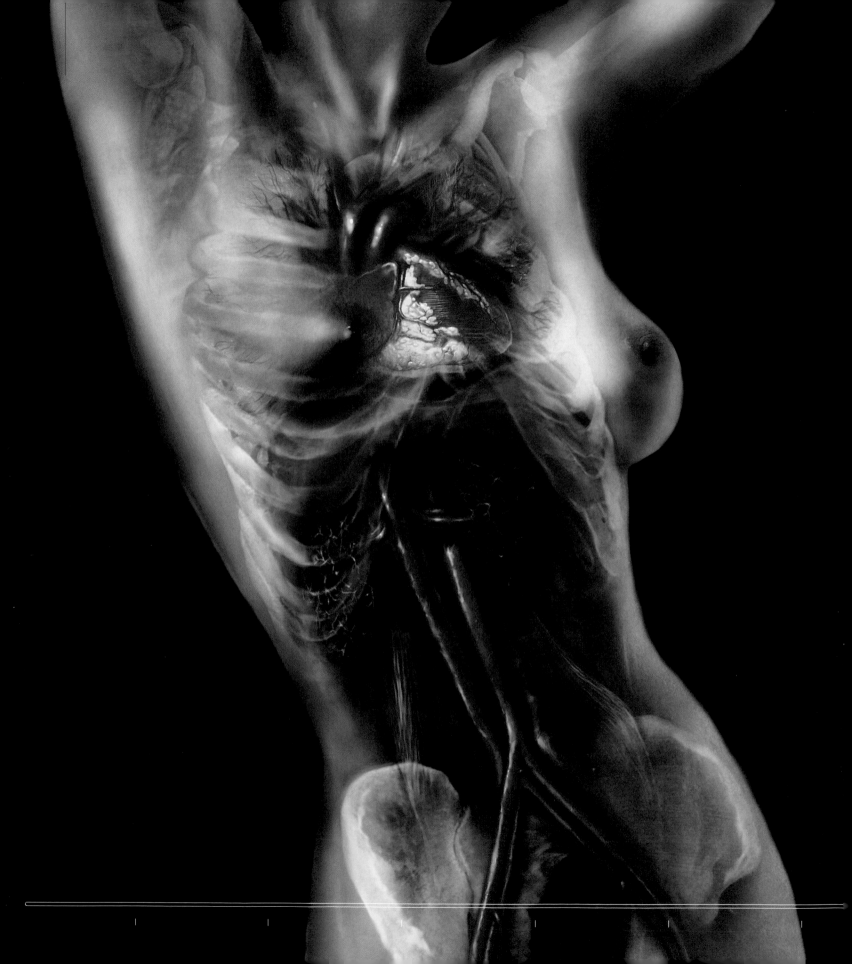

"EVERYTHING IS THE WAY IT IS BECAUSE IT GOT THAT WAY."

—D'ARCY THOMPSON

On a night in 1879, a raging North Sea gale knocked out the central spans of the world's longest bridge—the railway bridge at Dundee, Scotland— 2 miles of lattice girders supported by slender cast-iron columns and braced with wrought-iron struts and ties. The Industrial Revolution had made such mighty structures possible, by harnessing steam power in order to mold and mass-produce versatile new building materials, and the engineering prowess of the British railway system was unrivaled. When the spans were swept away, 75 passengers and crew on a passing train fell more than 100 feet into a freezing estuary and died, sending shock waves through the British engineering profession and the public at large.

The disaster—resulting a year later in the construction nearby of a new type of steel-and-masonry bridge, engineered to withstand just about anything—radically influenced the fields of architecture and design. Bridges, like buildings and turbines, are machines; they're built to do a job. By the end of the nineteeth century, the Machine Age—with its steel frames, reinforced concrete, electric elevators, curtain walling, and unprecedented opportunities for catastrophic failure—challenged architects to design functional structures out of new substances, in new ways, and for new purposes. Structural integrity became key; overbuilding, for reasons of liability if not always for safety, the norm.

The Tay Bridge collapse, and the bridge's replacement by the mighty Firth of Forth, also, as it turns out, shook up the study of *living* forms. In the decades since Charles Darwin had brilliantly concluded that such forms change through adaptation, few late-Victorian biologists hadn't turned their attention to *ancestry*: anatomical zoologists viewed bodily structures as archives evolving, like limbs from fish fins, out of previous forms. But D'Arcy Thompson, a broad-thinking Scot who soon arrived to teach college biology in Dundee, thought differently. Descended from Vikings, over 6 feet tall, regal in carriage, unpardonably handsome, D'Arcy (as he was always to be known) was a striding figure and dazzling conversationalist who, besides being a distinguished naturalist, was also an eminent Greek and Latin scholar, as well as a world-class mathematician. While scouting for shells and bones in the salt marshes out of which towered the greatest new engineering marvel of the era, his unusual blend of intellect and interests set him toward the more radical idea, expounded brilliantly over 60 years in books and articles, that living forms are hammered into shape not just through the endless adjustment of evolution, but from the combined action of physical forces—tension, compression, and shear. D'Arcy argued that the secret of life isn't heredity: it's engineering. Math and physics.

Take the problem of spanning 2 points—whether on the surface of a skin cell, from an ankle to a knee, or across the Mississippi. Unlike spans for transporting people and carriages, railway bridges must be rigid enough to carry the weight of locomotives and trains; suspension bridges are too supple. The solution? A cantilever bridge. The Forth Bridge is made of a pair of balanced arms—beams—that stick out like tightrope walkers' poles from 2 main towers and join at the middle. The beams are trussed with crisscrossing steel tubes, some up to 12 feet across, projecting diagonally from the tops and bottoms of the towers and fitted with internal stiffeners.

Built to carry loaded trains almost 300 yards from the nearest support, the bridge is one of the strongest (and most expensive) ever built. Its profile resembles a chain of stegosaurus skeletons—lumbering, squat-legged, humpbacked.

D'Arcy examined the rigging of Scotland's massive steel and stone bridges, and saw a diagram in the sky of the forces they were built to withstand. His naturalist's imagination came ablaze as he saw these mechanical structures mirrored up and down and throughout the realm of biology, of life. "In a suspension bridge," he wrote in his 1917 masterwork, *On Growth and Form*, "a great part of the fabric is subject to tensile strain only, and is built throughout of ropes and wires; but the massive piers at either end of the bridge carry the weight of the whole structure and its load, and endure all the 'compression strains' which are inherent in the system. Very much the same is the case in that wonderful arrangement of struts and ties which constitute, or complete, the skeleton of an animal."

A living skeleton is a marvel of mechanical efficiency, not at all like the jangly, immobilized museum pieces scientists wire and clamp together to keep them from crumpling in a heap. As D'Arcy observed, "ligament and membrane, muscle and tendon, run between bone and bone; and the beauty and strength of the mechanical construction lie not in one part or in another, but in the harmonious concatenation which all the parts, soft and hard, rigid and flexible, tension bearing and pressure bearing, make up together."

D'Arcy built his theory bottom-up, starting with the nonpliable cellular material that comprises the skeletal framework—what we call bone. From an engineer's standpoint, he wrote, "bone may seem weak indeed, but it has the great advantage of being nearly as good for a tie as for a strut, nearly as strong to withstand rupture, or tearing asunder, as to resist crushing." D'Arcy showed that live bone tissue, which normally we hope never to see, turns out to be as much of an engineering marvel as the skeleton itself—on the microscopic level. Bone is an intricate microstructure of hollow fibers: tubes. On its dense surface the tubes are compacted, but the interior is spongy. An irregular honeycomb of slender beams allows space in between for the manufacture of cells and storage of minerals, while also bracing the tube against being crushed, snapped, or pulled apart. As a building material, bone is stronger yet lighter than steel, and D'Arcy observed that the reason for this is the precise, efficient gridwork of the stabilizing tubes, which are arrayed at the exact angles and proper lengths to provide optimal strength and stability.

He wrote gleefully in *On Growth and Form* about "the great engineer, Professor Culmann of Zurich," who in 1866 had been consumed with the problem of designing a new and powerful crane.

Karl Culmann visited a colleague's dissecting room, where the anatomist was "contemplating the section of a bone":

> The engineer . . . saw in a moment that the arrangement of the bony trabeculae (micro-tubes) was nothing more or less than a diagram of the lines of stress, or directions of tension and compression, in the loaded structure: in short that nature was strengthening the bone in precisely the manner and direction in which strength was required; and he is said to have cried out, "that's my crane!"

D'Arcy mapped the web of stress lines in a human femur to illustrate Culmann's point. Looking something like the knobbed head of a walking stick, the femur is the forward of the 2 long tubes connecting the ankle and the knee—one of the longest and most vulnerable bones in the human body. The femur bears most of the body's full weight when standing, so it shouldn't surprise us that its gnarled, notched crown, unsymmetrical neck, and tapered length distribute the stress efficiently to keep it from buckling. D'Arcy's stress lines coincided exactly with the lattice formed naturally by the trabeculae. In a similar experiment, he examined the bone structure of a vulture's wing and found "a perfect Warren's truss, just as one as is often used for a main rib in an aeroplane."

Ultimately, it was the larger design of the Forth Bridge that inspired D'Arcy's crowning application of Machine Age engineering principles to the problem of living forms. "It is plain that each bone plays a part in relation to the whole body, analogous to that which a little trabecula, or a little group of trabeculae, plays within the bone itself," he wrote. In other words, in the job of making a skeleton that carries the full weight of an animal, nature arranged the bony tubes and straplike sinews into an optimal framework. Think of a quadruped, D'Arcy said: a horse in a standing posture. Chiefly, the bones serve as struts (in mechanical design terms, upright or sloping timbers), while the muscles and ligaments act as ties—cross-braces. Standing foursquare on its front and hind legs, with the weight of its body and maybe a rider suspended in between, the horse suggests a bridge "carried by its two piers."

But what type of bridge? The horse's curved backbone appears to be a simple arch, but it can't truly act as an arch unless it's held back at both ends, and the jointed legs give out too easily for that purpose. Nor do we see, as we do in some bridges, the addition of a lattice on the underside of the arch to tie the ends together, or a straight tie across, holding it like a bowstring. So what then? "The structure," D'Arcy wrote triumphantly, "is strictly and beautifully comparable to the main girder of a double armed cantilever bridge."

D'Arcy had found in the great coal-blackened wonders of pre–World War I England—the birthplace of the modern world—a new way of looking at life. Living forms, he believed, are inseparable from their functions: indeed, just like bridges, they are "diagrams" of the forces that hold them together. He agreed with Darwin that adaptation accounted for much, but insisted that, more than ancestry, *architecture*—mathematical forces—would ultimately explain more about how animate nature arises.

In his lifetime—D'Arcy died in 1948—most biologists dismissed him as a vastly learned and erudite, even brilliant, amateur. Limited to slide rules, scalpels, microscopes, and X rays, nobody could begin to critically evaluate, much less expand, on his work. "The mathematics available to D'Arcy Thompson could not prove what he wanted to prove," science writer James Gleick wrote in *Chaos*; neither could the revolution in biology, which "passed him by utterly." And so for most of the twentieth century, *On Growth and Form* was read more widely by people interested in designing new physical structures—architects and engineers—than by those concerned with the world inside us.

Until the past 75 years or so, those most concerned with that world, medical men and a few women, had only the most primitive tools and insights to guide their work. A year after *On Growth and Form* was published in Great Britain, the 1918 flu epidemic—one of the 3 deadliest contagions in history—killed 22 million people around the globe, nearly twice as many as died in World War I. The flu itself was not the killer; with no antibiotics or other treatments available, the victims' lungs became saturated with pneumonia-causing bacteria, and many died less than 48 hours after their first cough. To many people, the larger problem was scientific medicine itself. Though the germ theory of disease had been widely accepted for more than a generation, the actual mechanisms of immunity were unknown and unknowable. The Machine Age was roaring. Skyscrapers and airplanes heralded an era built upon mechanical structures far more complex and daring—more lifelike—than the steel bridges of the previous century. Yet medicine offered only palliatives—aspirin and minerals. "Science," the *New York Times* editorialized, "has failed to guard us."

Doctors and other scientists began to address this failure by delving deeper into the world of cells, the structural units of nearly every living thing. Cells perform different jobs and, as with buildings and machines, are constructed according to what they do. It had been an American architect, Louis Sullivan, so-called "Father of the Skyscraper," who first famously asserted that "form follows function" in a famous 1896 manifesto proclaiming the interconnection of utility and beauty in tall buildings. What Sullivan meant was that the design of a structure should faithfully reflect its purpose. Now, as scientists began to puzzle out the flu's dynamics—what caused it; how it spread so fast and killed so many—they applied the same principle to the cellular world.

For example, red blood cells load up with oxygen molecules in the lungs and exchange them with depleted tissue cells that, in return, hand over metabolic slag—junk minerals and gasses. They're microscopic ferries; their 2 main jobs involve picking up and dropping off small molecules. In contrast, the primary function of muscle cells is contraction. Bundled into ropelike cables equipped with armlike cross-bridges that bend, detach, straighten, and then repeat the process, billions of muscle cells hauling in unison can raise a finger, or an arm. As temporary grunt labor, healthy red blood cells have no need for nuclei; highly coordinated muscle cells, some measuring up to a foot long, can have many.

In 1926, two years before the British microbiologist Alexander Fleming accidentally discovered penicillin while trying to identify the microbe that caused the 1918 flu pandemic, a Swedish chemist named Theodor Svedberg built the first ultracentrifuge, a machine that, spinning at high revolution, can hurl matter outward at up to 1 million times the force of gravity. The device gave cellular biologists their first opportunity not only to separate cells from each other but to sift parts of a cell from the whole—based solely on their shape and size—and Svedberg received the Nobel Prize for his work. In fact, what he had done was to make it possible to examine the structural components inside cells—"organelles," which bear the same relation to cells as tissues to organs and organs to bodies. If, like bones and skeletons, these tiny forms were diagrams of the forces and interplays that defined their work, and if their construction determined what they did and how, perhaps engineering was the key to life after all.

Mitochondria, so-called "powerhouses" of the cell, contain the main molecular machinery for breaking down sugars and converting them into currents of energy—their mechanisms drive all living activity. Biologists long knew of their existence but couldn't begin studying them until the mid-1930s, when Svedberg's machines made it possible to isolate mitochondria from the other mini-organs packed inside the cell membrane. Using electron microscopes, invented in 1931 and offering resolutions measured in billionths of an inch, researchers observed that these infinitesimal reactors are generally spherical, with an outer membrane surrounding an inner membrane folded into scaffolding. The spongy lattice allows perfectly for what amounts to a molecular recycling plant, while giving support to the domelike structure around it—similar to the tubelike trabeculae in bone. Cells with the most metabolic activity, like those of the heart, not surprisingly were found to have the most fully developed mitochondria.

The quest to diagram the most basic living forms unleashed explosions in both biology and architecture,

as nearing mid-century the 2 converged at the same guiding idea: "function presupposes structure," as D'Arcy called it. What a thing does dictates its design. An apprentice to Louis Sullivan, Frank Lloyd Wright, began advocating for what he called "organic architecture"—buildings in which all parts are related to each other and to their site. Tired of being "the pencil in Sullivan's hand," Wright went on to help reformulate modern architecture for the Machine Age much as the engineer Alexandre-Gustave Eiffel had done following the Industrial Revolution, generating iconic new structures drawn from living shapes. Meanwhile, in 1927, 32-year-old Buckminster Fuller, then a bankrupt and discredited architect and inventor, whose first child had died and who verged on suicide, resolved to spend his life developing what he called "Comprehensive Anticipatory Design Science." Following D'Arcy's lead, Fuller believed there existed a universal "geometry of energy" that existed throughout nature, regular patterns linking man-devised structures like frames, trusses, and buildings to the behavior of molecules and atoms. Fuller's most famous creation, the geodesic dome, is the lightest, strongest, most cost-effective shelter ever designed. As he proudly explained, it derives its shape from cells and organelles.

It was after World War II that the defining advances in the study of the human body began to reflect more fully D'Arcy's structure-based point of view. The first half of the twentieth century was dominated scientifically by the physicists, mathematicians, and cosmologists who broke the secrets of the atom. Now, quantum physics revolutionized the study of life itself, while giving scientists powerful new tools to deconstruct living forms at every level—molecule, cell, tissue, organ, system, and organism.

In 1948, the year D'Arcy died, the American chemist Linus Pauling claimed he was lying in bed with a bad cold when he happened on a structure—a spiral, or helix—that could explain how some long chains of atoms folded together to form proteins, the functional molecules in cells. Proteins are complex, twisting, convoluted, *active* molecules—the industrial machinery of the molecular world. Yet the distance between their components is measured in billionths of a meter and they act in milliseconds. With just pencils and slide rules to compute the forces and dynamics of their chemical interactions, and borrowing the architect's craft of building scale models, Pauling's lab demonstrated how molecules fold and refold using the same few structural components—coils, corkscrews, chains and side chains, threads, and "pleated sheets."

After publishing his results in 1951, Pauling turned his attention to solving the structure of another type of biologically active molecule—the nucleic acids. During World War II, the exiled German theoretical physicist Erwin Schrödinger proposed that genetic information life's blue prints—must be stored at the atomic level. A year later, an American bacteriologist, Oswald Avery, found that an extract of DNA from dead germs could "transform" healthy ones. Pauling, later a 2-time solo winner of the Nobel Prize (for chemistry and peace), was closing in on the molecule's structure when, in 1953, he was famously bested by 2 unknown scientists in England, Francis Crick and James Watson, and their collaborators. Borrowing from physics, researchers had now learned to "solve" the structures of simple molecules by bombarding them with X rays and measuring how the beams diffracted. Using such visual data, Watson and Crick were able to build from tubes and strips of cardboard a model of DNA that looked like a gently spiraling ladder. The "secret of life," as Watson triumphantly called it, turned out to be a right-handed spiral staircase, an architectural motif believed to have been first used in medieval castles, where tower staircases corkscrewed counterclockwise to give right-handed swordsmen an advantage in stabbing intruders.

Schrödinger's assertions also captivated the visionary mathematician Alan Turing. Best known as the eccentric young code breaker who helped England crack Nazi U-boat codes, and as the father of the digital computer, Turing also pioneered a novel approach for probing life's deepest structures. As a Cambridge don before the war, Turing invented the world's first "thinking machine," both as an attempt to replicate the logical processes of the human brain and as a tool to help answer a basic question about life, one that had enthralled him ever since he was a lonely 12-year-old: How does anything *know* how to grow? Turing understood that as cells divide, they differentiate, organizing themselves into complex structures—tissues—which coordinate with other structures to form organs and, ultimately, biological systems. Life was an endless process of one thing developing—morphing—into another. Yet change required force, direction. For Turing, Schrödinger's speculations about genes centered around a chemical—*structural*—question: How was the information in genes translated into action? What were the mathematical principles underlying the chemistry of life?

In 1952, he proposed an answer. Using one of the first primitive computers, a gargantuan contraption of electrical switches that he directed like an organ master at a huge keyboard, Turing analyzed the coat patterns of mammals and discerned an underlying set of linear equations. In this instance he showed convincingly that life *was* math—something to be puzzled out by examining the forces inherent in molecular reactions—in much the same way that D'Arcy had puzzled out the dynamics of animal skeletons by looking at stress lines. Turing proposed a process he called "morphogenesis," in which certain genes signal others where to go in order to build an organism from the inside out, dictating the size and shape of structures at every level. And he posited the existence of morphogens—genes that carry and relay the blueprints for building living structures. Nature's foremen, in other words. (After being arrested on charges of homosexuality and forced by the British government to take masculine hormones, Turing killed himself in 1954, just as his work in computers and insights into biology were catching up with each other.)

Work on morphogens languished after Turing's death, even as new approaches flourished for *visualizing* what goes on inside living things. D'Arcy saw skeletons as bridges, but no one at the time could look inside the deepest structures of a living brain or a heart valve or a 10-day-old human embryo or a hemoglobin molecule. By the fifties, however, that began to change. Nuclear physicists had known since the thirties that spinning atomic particles wobble at a characteristic frequency, like billions of infinitesimal children's tops tilting in unison. In 1952, the Nobel Prize in physics went to 2

Americans, Felix Bloch and Edward Purcell, for their discovery of "nuclear magnetic resonance." What Bloch and Purcell found, working independently of each other, is that powerful magnets can force the particles to "flip"—change frequency—and that by studying the process you could investigate the physical structure of matter. The discovery laid the groundwork for magnetic resonance imaging, or MRI, which enabled researchers to examine the inside of soft tissue, even the brain.

In 1959, after 12 years of painstaking assembly, 2 pioneering English biochemists solved the first three-dimensional structure of a protein molecule. Under optimal conditions, proteins crystallize—in effect, freeze in a continuous matrix. By beaming crystallized whale hemoglobin with X rays and examining how the beams diffracted, Max Perutz and John Kendrew found that the molecule is composed of 4 separate chains of atoms, each exposing an iron-based compound at the surface. The 4-part architecture is common in botany—showing up, for instance, in the sepals, petals, and stamens of the evening primrose—and iron-based groups optimally placed to pick up, transport, and release oxygen molecules. Perutz and Kendrew shared the 1962 Nobel Prize for chemistry.

Molecular assembly—not composition—now became "the central and most productive question in modern chemistry," according to chronicler Howard Freeland Judson. The term "structural biology" started to refer almost exclusively to the behavior of large molecules in cells. Then, by the late 1970s, the structure-based revolution in chemistry also overtook biology, especially medicine; increasingly, doctors began to view disease as a mechanical process, and drug researchers studied the structural interaction of molecules for clues about how to make better drugs.

Meanwhile, the heirs to Turing's thinking machines pushed nuclear medicine dramatically ahead with the introduction of computerized tomography (CT) and other scanning techniques. Invented in England by a radiologist named Gedfrey Hounsfield, who also won a Nobel Prize for his work, CT involves surveying the body with X rays from several angles simultaneously, then measuring the beams' strength after they've passed through. Beams that pass through dense tissue such as bone—or a solid tumor—will be weaker than those that pass through, say, lung tissue. The result: the ability to generate multiple cross-sections throughout the body.

With MRIs and computers and CT scans, and other new tools such as ultrasound, doctors near the end of the millennium were able to do what chemists and biologists had been doing at the molecular level for decades: generate 3-D views of hidden structures. (Architects had meanwhile begun to use comparable technologies to take apart and reassemble conventional boxlike buildings into shapelier, more lifelike new forms, such as Frank Gehry's iconic, billowing, titanium-sheathed Guggenheim Museum in Bilbao, Spain.) Further, the explosion in genomics—and in developmental biology, which looks at how living forms take shape—began to reveal the ultimate mystery behind the forms: growth. How does anything know how to grow? Alan Turing had asked. The answer: by the secretion of "signaling" molecules, which chemically position other molecules as they assemble themselves into active forms. That is, by morphogens, as Turing had predicted in 1952.

Modern science has lately begun to catch up with D'Arcy's claims that the chemistry of life is based on mathematical theory, and that math and physics can explain the shapes living things take and how they take them. The tools to "prove what he wanted to prove" no longer lag behind; indeed, their exploratory potential now seems boundless. Recently, a NASA scientist looking for evidence of life on Mars devised an intelligent software system. Running on thousands of computers networked through the Internet, David Noever's program spends its time combing through billions of images—photos of cross-sections of meteorites scoured from the Antarctic ice—looking for microscopic fossils. It scans for signature shapes or patterns that are only observed when there are cells present—in other words, the shapes of life. To honor the pioneer who inspired it—and with a nod to Turing—Noever has named his vast artificial neural network "The D'Arcy Machine."

....

"MAN IS THE
MEASURE OF ALL THINGS."
— PROTAGORAS (490–420 B.C.E.)

....

The desire to explore our inner cosmos dates back to ancient times. Aristotle, who dissected 400 species of plants and animals but never a human, argued that every organ has its own function, which can be deduced from its structure. Some of his deductions missed their mark—he believed the seat of the mind was the heart, for example—but his linkage of form and function has governed anatomical studies ever since. A century after his death, the Egyptian Herophilus performed the first recorded human dissections.

During the Renaissance, the study of human anatomy produced a "culture of dissection," which, as historian Jonathan Sawday notes, helped both to stir up the imaginative arts—poetry, drama, painting, sculpture, and, above all, architecture—and to popularize the notion of a "mechanical body." This new conception arose mainly from the work of Leonardo da Vinci, who in the 1490s began his anatomical studies by taking apart machines and studying what he called their "organs"—screws, pulleys, chains, ropes, belts, axles, bearings, springs, cams, crankshafts, flywheels, transmission systems, and shock absorbers. In 1510, he turned his attention to humans, "passing the night in the company of . . . corpses, quartered, flayed and terrible to behold," he wrote. Resorting to innovative graphic techniques such as "see-through" images, exploded views, drawings from different vantage points, and the depiction of muscles as lines of force, he revealed a towering complexity. Like Aristotle, he was limited by the available science; he stuck to the traditional view that nerves were tubes carrying airflows that caused muscles to contract by inflation. But his meticulous investigations raised dissection to the level of art. Throughout Europe, dissection became fashionable as the curious and well-to-do flocked to "anatomy theaters," where stolen cadavers were "emblazoned" and lectured upon.

Each subsequent age has built on the Renaissance metaphor of the "mechanical body," revealing something of how it views its new technological and social realities (and reflecting its archi-

tectural and design concepts). The Industrial Age of a century and a half ago yielded the view that the human interior resembled not just a machine, but also a *factory*—an automated combine of complex mechanical wonders. With the introduction of electricity a few decades later, systems—power grids, transportation and communication networks, organizational matrices—revolutionized modern life. The body was then compared to a corporation, with the brain the central office, the peripheral nervous system a telephone network connecting far-flung activities, the bloodstream contributing supply and distribution lines, and so forth. During the Atomic Age that followed, the body became at once more molecular and more universal. The 1966 science fiction thriller *Fantastic Voyage* told the story: A team of scientists, shrunk to the size of viruses so they can be injected into the bloodstream of a wounded nuclear scientist, journey through the body's myriad cavities, where they dodge the clinging death-grip of chainlike antibodies and breach greasy cell walls to fix a remote area of the brain. A decade later, at the height of the Space Age, the metaphors were extraterrestrial: "The blastocyst has landed!" *Life* magazine trumpeted alongside photographs of an embryo implanting in its mother's uterus.

Depending on who's talking now, we live in either the Information Age or the Genomic Age. Both provide their own striking metaphors to suggest that the "mechanical body" of the past is now giving way to newer, more complex ways of viewing how we are built and what we are made of. Think of the Internet, the first man-made structure to approach the complexity of the human brain. Like Leonardo discovering the similarities between blood vessels, trees, and canals, or like D'Arcy comparing airplane wing trusses to bones, we understand that the human brain is heavily networked, and that its circuitry looks a lot like the World Wide Web. The architecture and design of the Internet is to today's neurologists what the engineering of the Forth Bridge was to D'Arcy—both a reflection of our deepest structures and a tool for understanding them. Similarly, the decoding of the Human Genome—described universally as our "blueprint"—has given science not only the understanding of how life is built, but the power to build it. Combine the Internet's lightning-like signaling power with DNA's ability to reproduce itself—and add new theories of math, such as Chaos, which discern order and pattern in seemingly random occurrences—and what you get is pretty close to the definition of intelligent life. Call it Infonomics.

To produce the landmark images in this book, artist Alexander Tsiaras has confronted the internal dimensions of the human figure with the core technologies of the Infonomic Age, and for the first time we see the body interior not as *like* something, or represented pictorially by human hands, or as a grainy negative or video image, but very nearly as it is. Reconstituting data from the full array of new body-scans, ultrapowerful microscopes, and molecular surveillance tools, Tsiaras conducts virtual dissections. His scalpel, so to speak, is an advanced graphics computer, upon which he composes not photographs—since photography is useful only with visible objects and can't penetrate surfaces that reflect light—but *visualizations*. Leonardo's "see-through" images, exploded views, and multiple vantage points allowed him to peel back layers of tissue

to expose what went on within us. Tsiaras, using software that allows him to pick apart the most delicate tissue or tiniest object, isolates structures that have never been seen before. Zooming in, he can rotate them in any direction, make them opaque if he likes. He has complete control over light and shadow, and his palette is limitless. The result: views so lifelike that metaphors may no longer be useful.

Dr. Oliver Wendell Holmes, Sr., in his 1858 poem "The Living Temple," also known as "The Anatomist's Hymn," rhapsodized about the flexible hidden architecture of bone, nerve, and brain that animates a human frame in motion: "Its living marbles jointed strong/With glistening band and silvery thong,/And linked to reason's guiding reins/By myriad rings in trembling chains." By the mid-nineteenth century, dissection had become primarily a teaching tool, and Holmes knew about "silvery thongs" of ligament and tendon and "trembling chains" of long nerves, because he had held them in his hands. Holmes's evocation of the body as a sacred building should come as no surprise. Nor, it turns out, should his stirring and erotic language: Anatomia, the Greek goddess of reductive division, was a woman. And as Sawday points out, the Renaissance culture of dissection was largely about sex, desire, and the thrill of the forbidden.

Tsiaras, happily for us, has followed in this tradition. The biological differences between men and women, it can be argued, animate life. Certainly they make it more interesting. By turning his tools and fascination toward the anatomical distinctions between males and females, Tsiaras has managed to reintroduce something else that all great explorations of the human body must include—but these days seldom do—an erotic frisson.

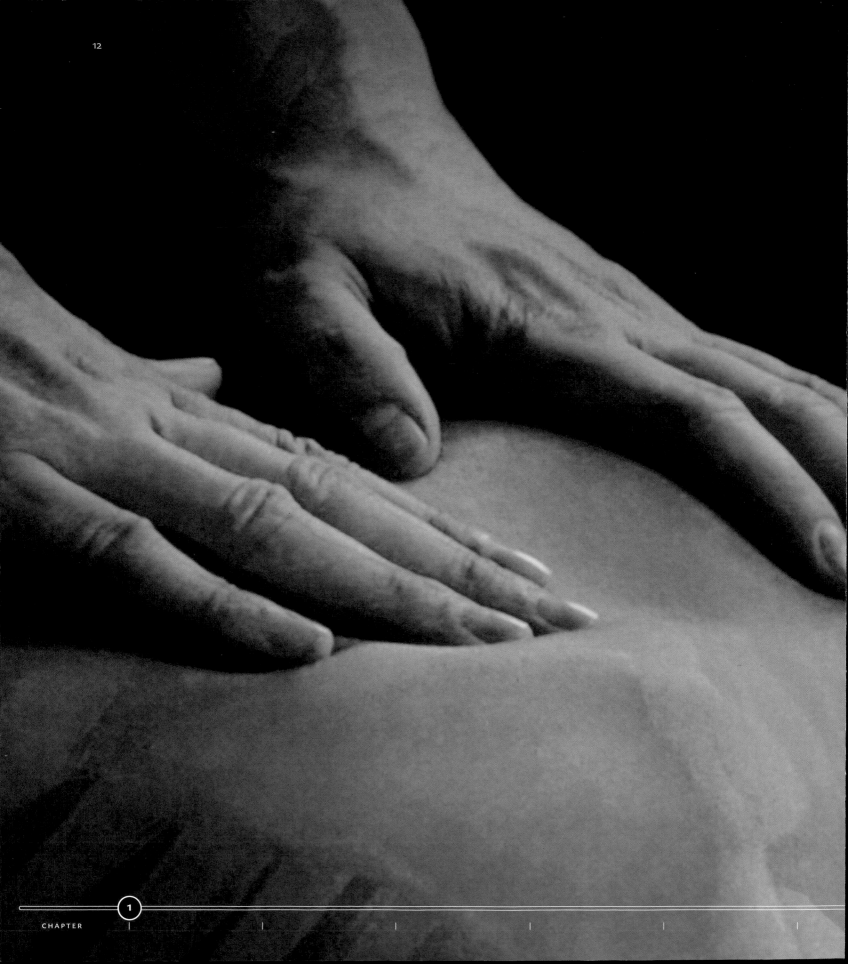

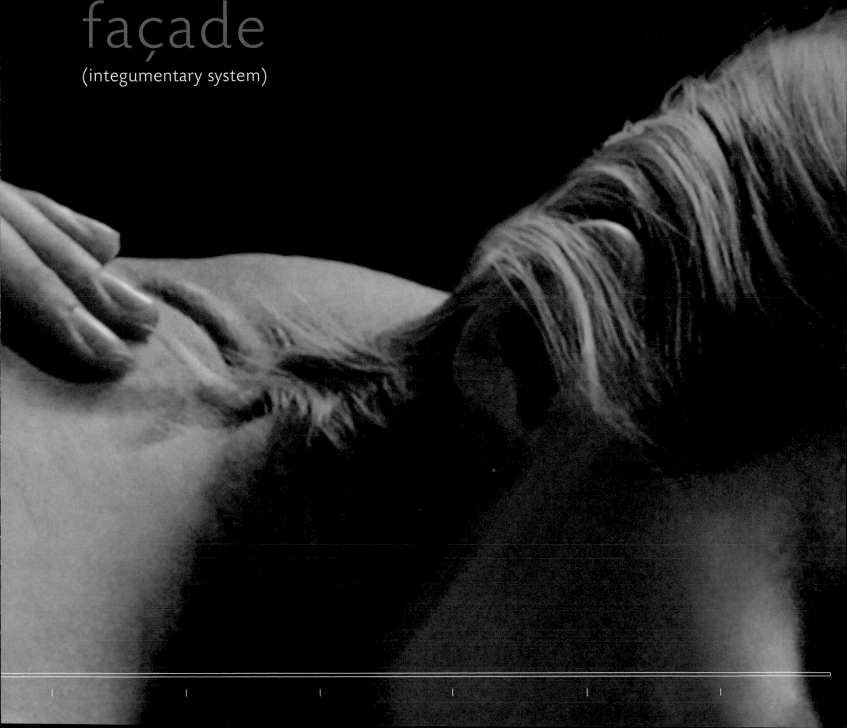

façade

(integumentary system)

Like other organs, the flesh and its appendages perform varied functions. Besides protecting us from damage due to physical injury, toxins, sunlight, heat, infection, and excessive water (and also from water loss), it maintains body temperature, detects physical sensation, produces Vitamin D, eliminates some waste materials, improves our grip of objects, and absorbs certain chemical substances. All this takes place within a pliant sheet of organic fabric studded with glands and hair follicles and filigreed with creases, grooves, ridges, and bumps; and ranges in thickness from $1/50$ inch in the eyelid to $1/6$ inch in the footsole—approximately the difference between fine angel-hair pasta and fettuccini.

A tough, semiporous laminate, skin is one of the largest structures in the body and consists of 2 distinct layers. The outer coating (epidermis) is a flexible, thin, semitransparent membrane of dead cells firmly dovetailed together (think of the surface of a blister bubble). The underlying base is a feltwork of fibrous and elastic tissue, the key structural element of which is keratin, a protein that also shows up in reptile scales (though not fish scales), bird feathers, claws, hooves, tooth enamel, horns (but not antlers), and hair. Keratin molecules twist around each other and contain sulfur, atoms of which are able to interlock with each other, rigidifying each twist.

Rubbery and elastic in infants, the system hardens and thickens with age, measuring in adulthood up to 2 square meters and weighing 10 to 12 pounds.

LIVING ENVELOPES

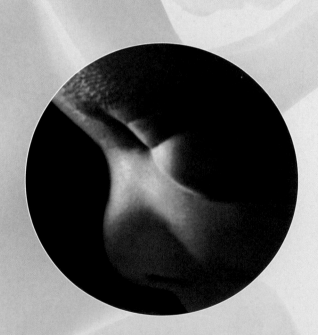

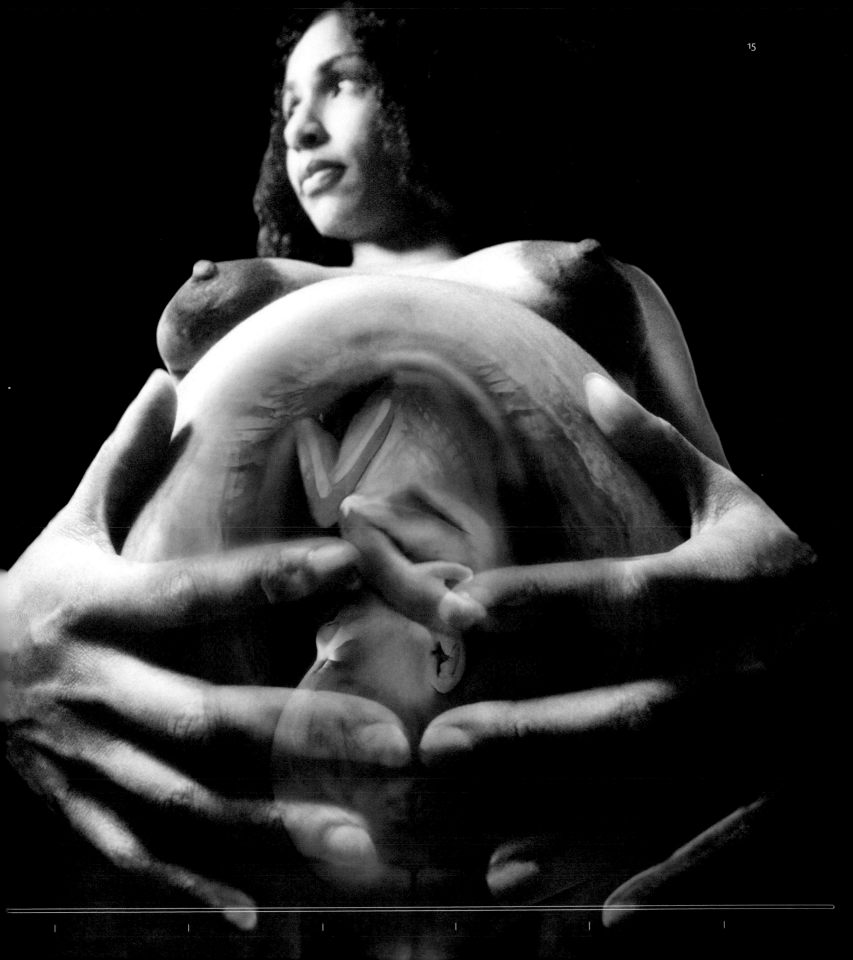

TOUGH YET SENSITIVE

The skin's underlying architecture varies according to location and activity, but continual resurfacing occurs throughout the life of the organ. Dead, flattened cells on the topmost layer are constantly worn away—most house dust is skin detritus—and replaced by new cells produced by the division of living cells at the base of the epidermis. The process takes about a month. As skin cells push up and move away from their source of nourishment, they flatten and shrink. As they move up to the "horny layer" at the surface, they lose their nuclei and turn into a lifeless protein—keratin. Keratin in the dead cells creates a tough, continuous fabric, its sulfur bonds too robust to be broken down by normal digestive enzymes. This prevents potentially invasive microbes from getting a purchase.

The inner dermis maintains its structural integrity, a fibrous tissue permeated with blood vessels, nerves, sweat and oil glands, and hair follicles, its deepest layer anchored to underlying tissues. Each square inch of skin houses about 700 sweat glands, 100 sebaceous or oil glands, and 21,000 sensors of heat, pressure, and pain.

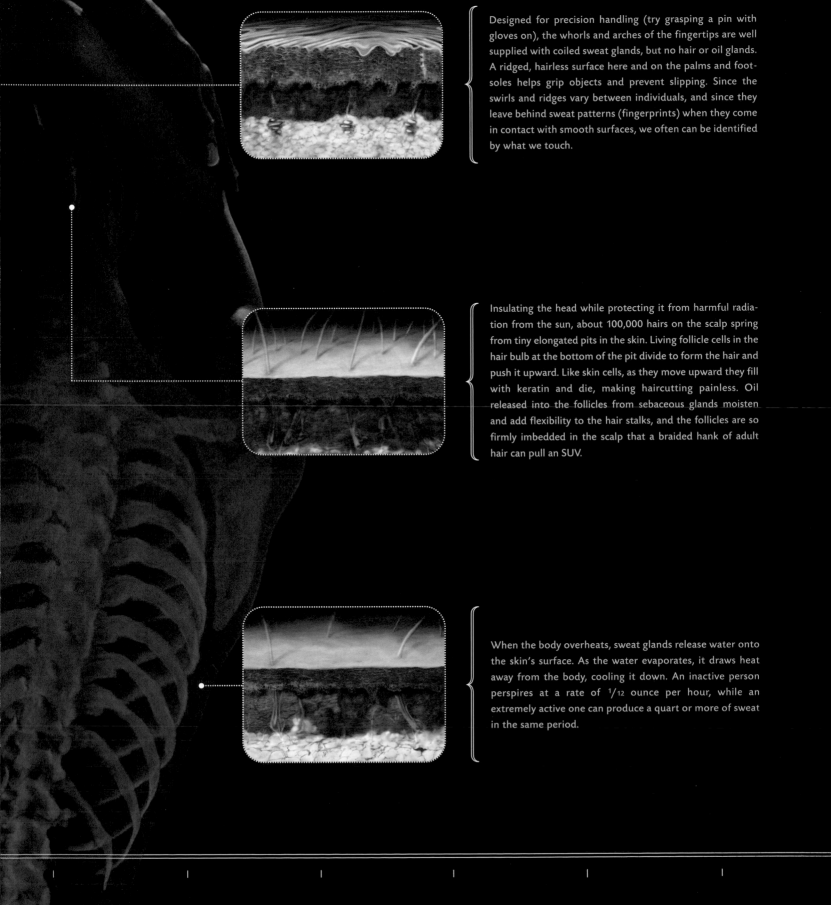

Designed for precision handling (try grasping a pin with gloves on), the whorls and arches of the fingertips are well supplied with coiled sweat glands, but no hair or oil glands. A ridged, hairless surface here and on the palms and foot-soles helps grip objects and prevent slipping. Since the swirls and ridges vary between individuals, and since they leave behind sweat patterns (fingerprints) when they come in contact with smooth surfaces, we often can be identified by what we touch.

Insulating the head while protecting it from harmful radiation from the sun, about 100,000 hairs on the scalp spring from tiny elongated pits in the skin. Living follicle cells in the hair bulb at the bottom of the pit divide to form the hair and push it upward. Like skin cells, as they move upward they fill with keratin and die, making haircutting painless. Oil released into the follicles from sebaceous glands moisten and add flexibility to the hair stalks, and the follicles are so firmly imbedded in the scalp that a braided hank of adult hair can pull an SUV.

When the body overheats, sweat glands release water onto the skin's surface. As the water evaporates, it draws heat away from the body, cooling it down. An inactive person perspires at a rate of $1/12$ ounce per hour, while an extremely active one can produce a quart or more of sweat in the same period.

Male and female exteriors, while functionally the same, differ in the production of skin oils and the distribution of hair and body fat. In other words, we deem physical appearance either as "masculine" or "feminine" less on the basis of sex than on specific patterns of development.

Men store body fat chiefly in the abdomen, women in the lower body, which becomes especially apparent in the different ways that we first fill out, then sag, as we age. Meanwhile, steroid hormones called androgens (testosterone is the best known)

GENDER DIFFERENCES

stimulate the production of sebum, a complex mixture of fats that causes hair to both coarsen and grow in a characteristically "male" configuration—face, chest, and abdomen. Since women also produce androgens, and men produce estrogens (hormones that stimulate "female" sexual characteristics), where, when, and what type of hairs we sprout is a composite of male and female patterns.

Hormones, not gender, are key. Women given testosterone shots develop male-pattern baldness while normal men often develop female-style hair loss.

MAN

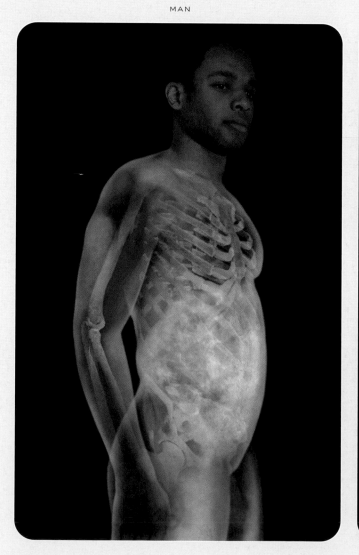

WOMAN

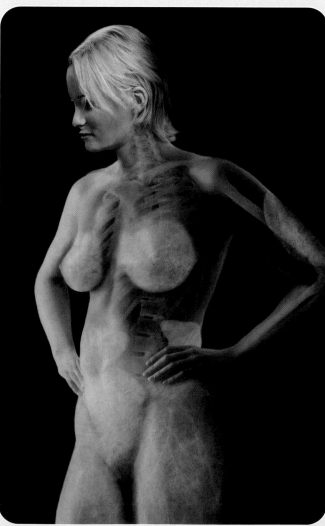

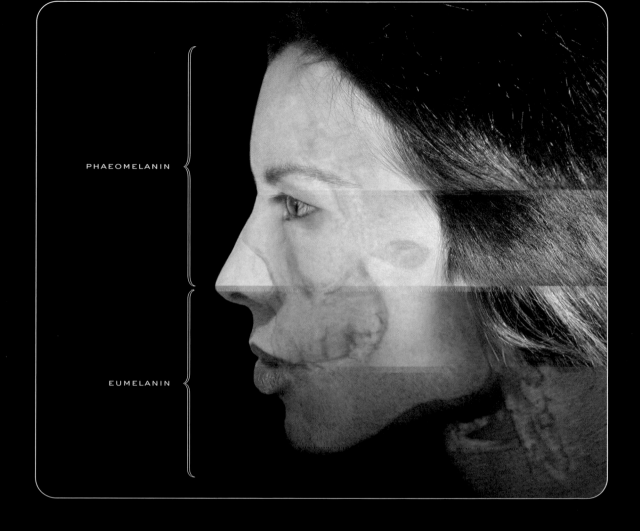

PHAEOMELANIN

EUMELANIN

A tanned skin is something more than respectable, and perhaps olive is a fitter color than white for a man—a denizen of the woods. "The pale white man!" I do not wonder that the African pitied him.

—Henry David Thoreau

The purpose of color in skin and hair supercedes vanity, identity, and other types of camouflage. Acting as a sunblock, the pigment melanin (yellow to red phaeomelanin, and dark-brown to black eumelanin) helps screen ultraviolet radiation, which, if let through, would damage the DNA in underlying tissues.

Tentacled cells called melanocytes stud the base of the epidermis, producing melanin and injecting it up into the layers of keratin-producing cells near the outer skin. Present throughout the body, melanocytes are most concentrated in the sex organs, nipples, armpits, and anal region, supplying extra protection for sensitive regions as well as attention-getting visual accents of use in the mating process.

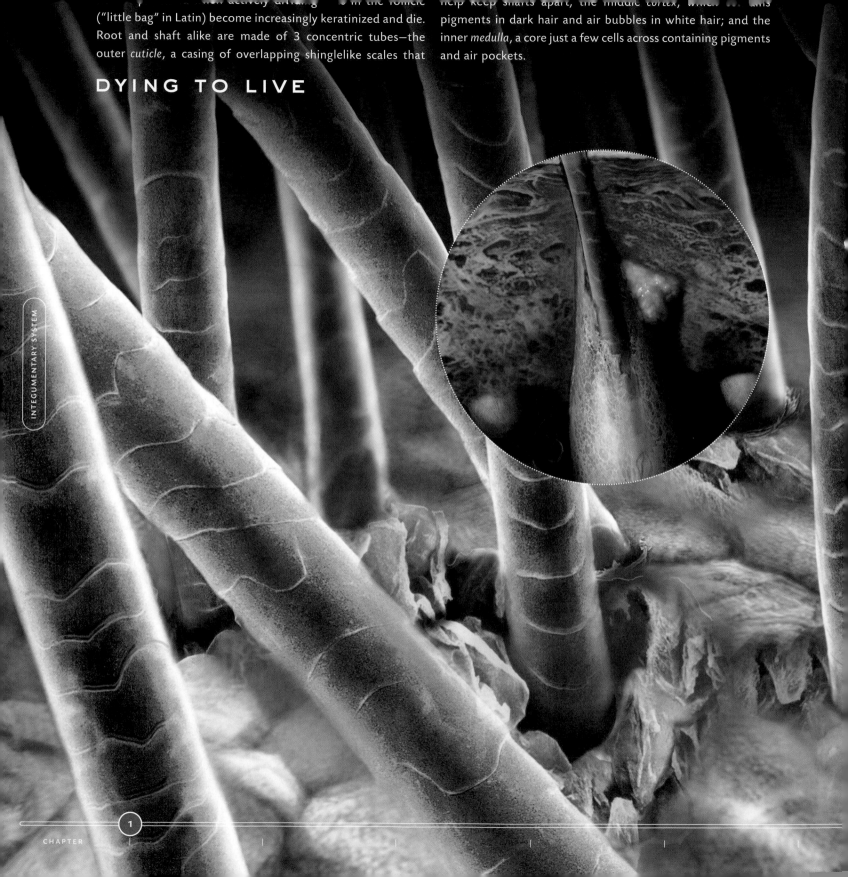

("little bag" in Latin) become increasingly keratinized and die. Root and shaft alike are made of 3 concentric tubes—the outer *cuticle*, a casing of overlapping shinglelike scales that

pigments in dark hair and air bubbles in white hair; and the inner *medulla*, a core just a few cells across containing pigments and air pockets.

DYING TO LIVE

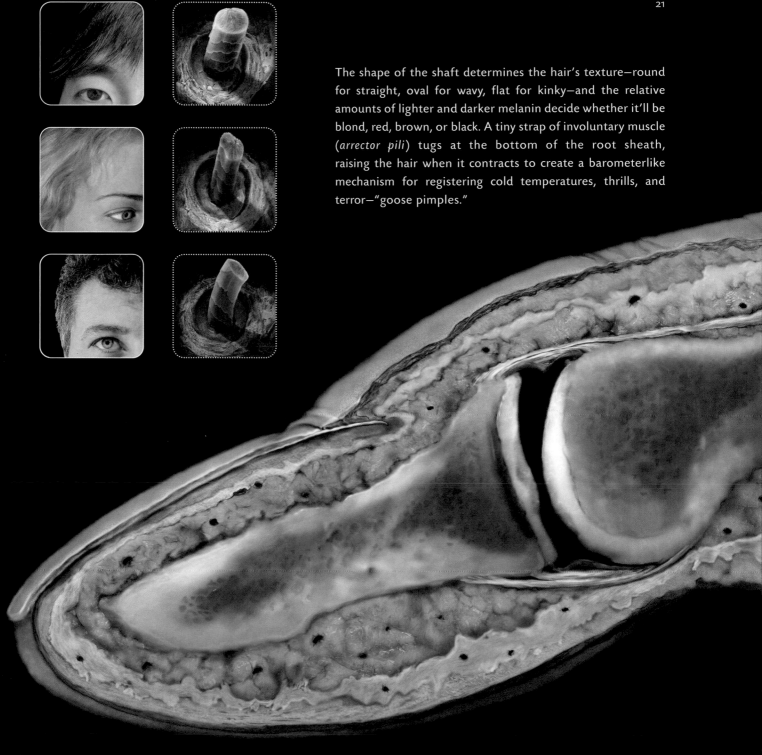

The shape of the shaft determines the hair's texture—round for straight, oval for wavy, flat for kinky—and the relative amounts of lighter and darker melanin decide whether it'll be blond, red, brown, or black. A tiny strap of involuntary muscle (*arrector pili*) tugs at the bottom of the root sheath, raising the hair when it contracts to create a barometerlike mechanism for registering cold temperatures, thrills, and terror—"goose pimples."

Guarding the ends of the fingers and toes, nails are hard plates of tightly packed keratinized cells. A hidden matrix of dividing epidermal cells beneath the root (visible as a white crescent at the base of the nail: the lunula) proliferates, pushing the plate forward. The nail bed, the portion of the nail we see, extends past the digit to the free edge, the distal part of the nail that needs to be clipped. Useful for grasping and scratching, nails grow faster in warm weather than cold, and fingernails grow 300 to 400 percent faster than toenails, a favorable ratio (and a relief to the back) since they're easier to clip.

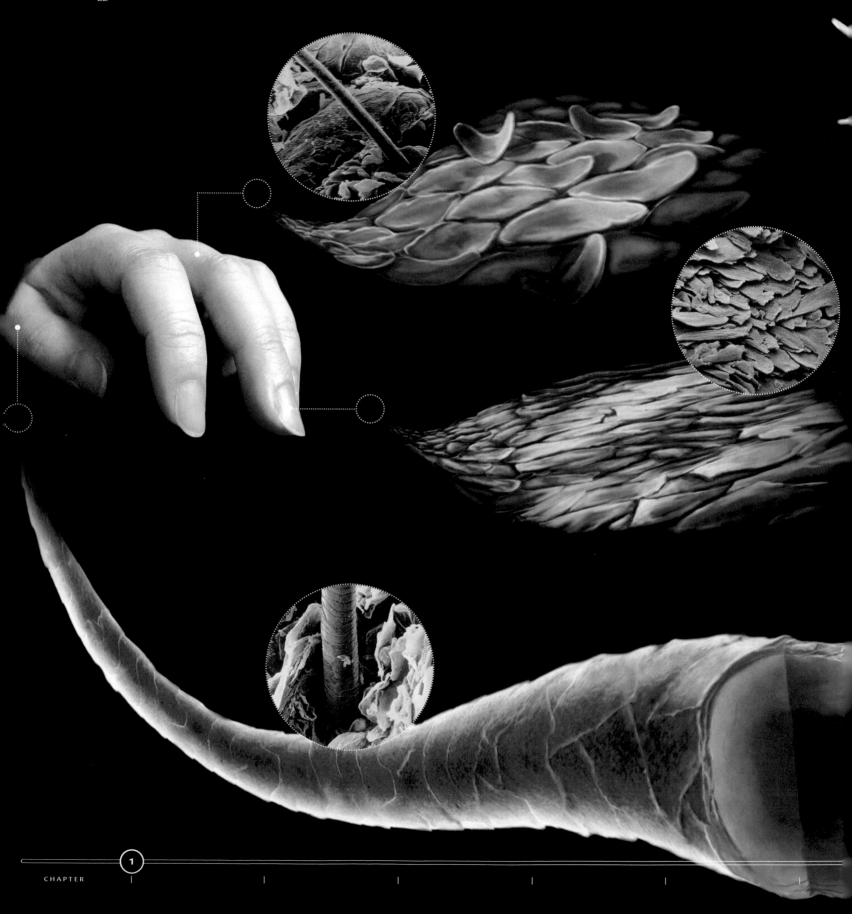

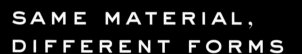

KERATIN PROTEIN ·······························●

SAME MATERIAL, DIFFERENT FORMS

Skin, hair, and nails are mostly protein. Keratin, like all working molecules in cells, is made of long chains of amino acids coiled like phone cords. But it's unique in that its chains contain high levels of sulfur atoms, which, when they come together, create one of the strongest chemical bonds in nature—disulphide linkages. The outer coating of a hair is comprised of dead keratinized cells, bundled lengthwise, their disulphide linkages tying the coils together like the rungs of a ladder.

Keratinized cells on the surface of the skin form tight, interlocking fan-shaped joints, weaving together into a rugged, tarplike fabric that keeps even microbes out and water and other essential substances in. In nails, they overlap like shingles, forging a clear, shell-like casing.

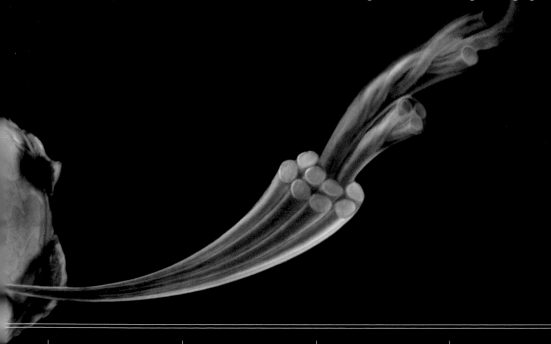

MIRRORED IN NATURE

Structurally, organic forms built from the same stuff and/or performing comparable jobs demonstrate a close likeness. The human epidermis resembles the bark of a maple tree. Shedding skin cells are compacted and corrugated like the collared heads of certain greens, allowing for surface expansion when what lies within bulges and eventually protrudes. Seedlings and hairs alike

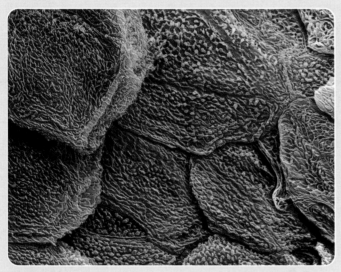

EPIDERMIS OF THE HAND

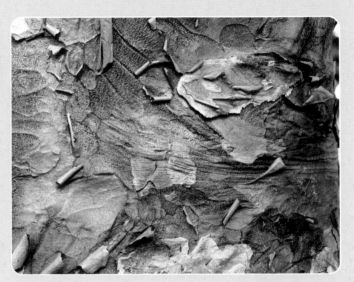

BARK OF MAPLE TREE

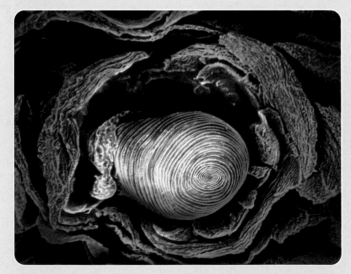

HAIR FOLLICLE EMERGING FROM TOPMOST LAYER OF
SHEDDING SKIN

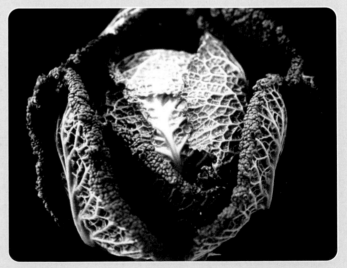

CABBAGE

unspool from saclike structures that nourish their growth. The thatch of keratin scales in a microscopic section of fingernail, for instance, stiffens the nail while protecting its underside, much like the scales of a silverfish.

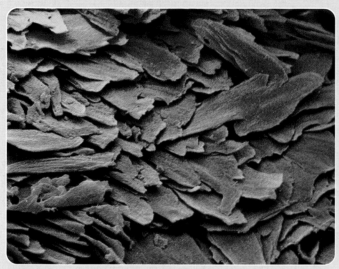

FINGER NAIL SURFACE

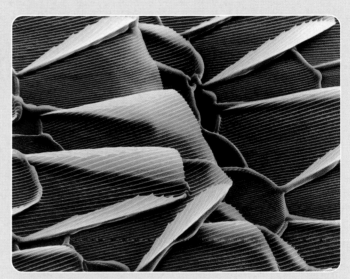

SCALES OF A SILVERFISH

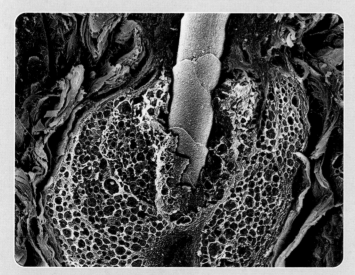

CROSS SECTION OF HAIR FOLLICLE

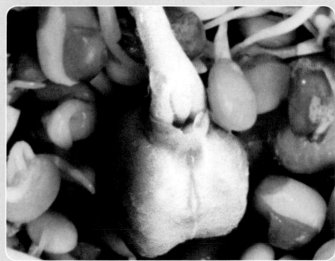

SPROUTING SEED

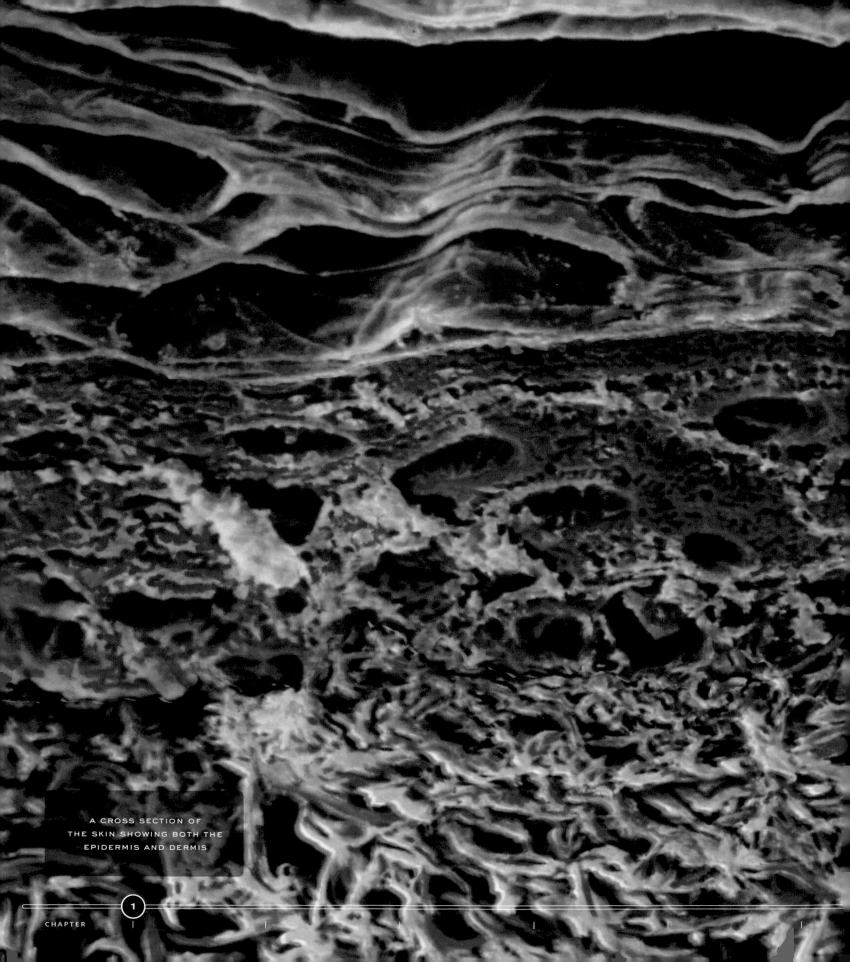

A CROSS SECTION OF
THE SKIN SHOWING BOTH THE
EPIDERMIS AND DERMIS

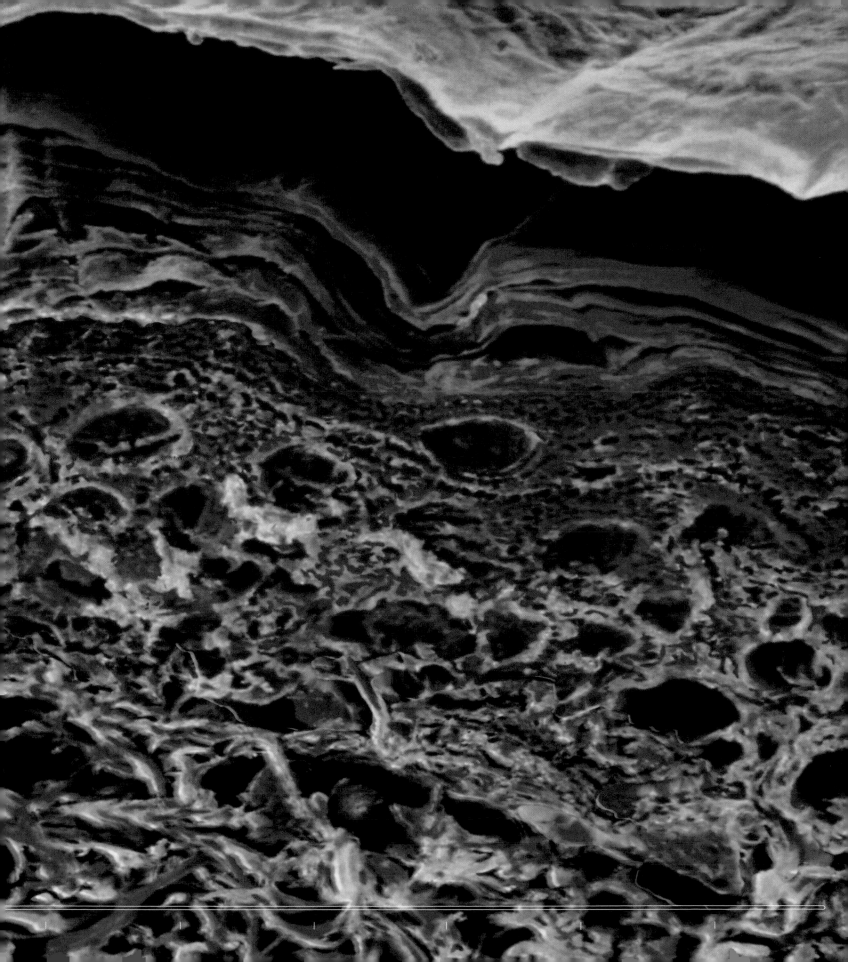

control–
electrochemical

(brain and nervous system)

Descartes meant the comparison. He understood all human action as reflexes: A stimulus excites a sense organ, which sends a message upward to the spinal cord or brain, which in turn relays the "excitation" downward to a muscle or gland, thus producing activity. He believed nerves were open tubes conveying tiny gusts of pressure throughout the body, much like the water pipes that made Renaissance fountains erupt in elaborate sequences. Descartes located the control center for these bursts of spirit—a kind of master switching station where all the tubes in and out of the brain ultimately converged—in the soul, which he said resided in the bean-sized pineal gland in the middle of the forebrain.

Why this and other theories of animal spiritus persisted as long as they did seems curious, since by Descartes' time anatomists had dissected human brains and nerves and discovered that they were made of fibers, not tubes. Yet it wasn't until the late eighteenth century that physiologists put together recent work on electricity and theories about the nervous system. Anatomists could trace the branching architecture of neural pathways, but the chemical and electrical signals animating them were beyond comprehension.

Not anymore. Neurologists and basic biologists, who see the nervous system as an ultra-high-speed communications network, have identified many of the electrochemical mechanisms at work. These include dozens of large molecules that convey signals within cells and from cell to cell, as well as newly discovered families of proteins (little nose cones) that guide nerve cells to make effective connections and others that hold all 100 billion neurons—the body's wiring—in place. Molecular glue, so to speak. The eminent Danish anatomist of Descartes' era who moaned, "The brain, the masterpiece of creation, is almost unknown to us," would be dazzled, although scientists and philosophers are probably no closer to locating a biological seat for the soul.

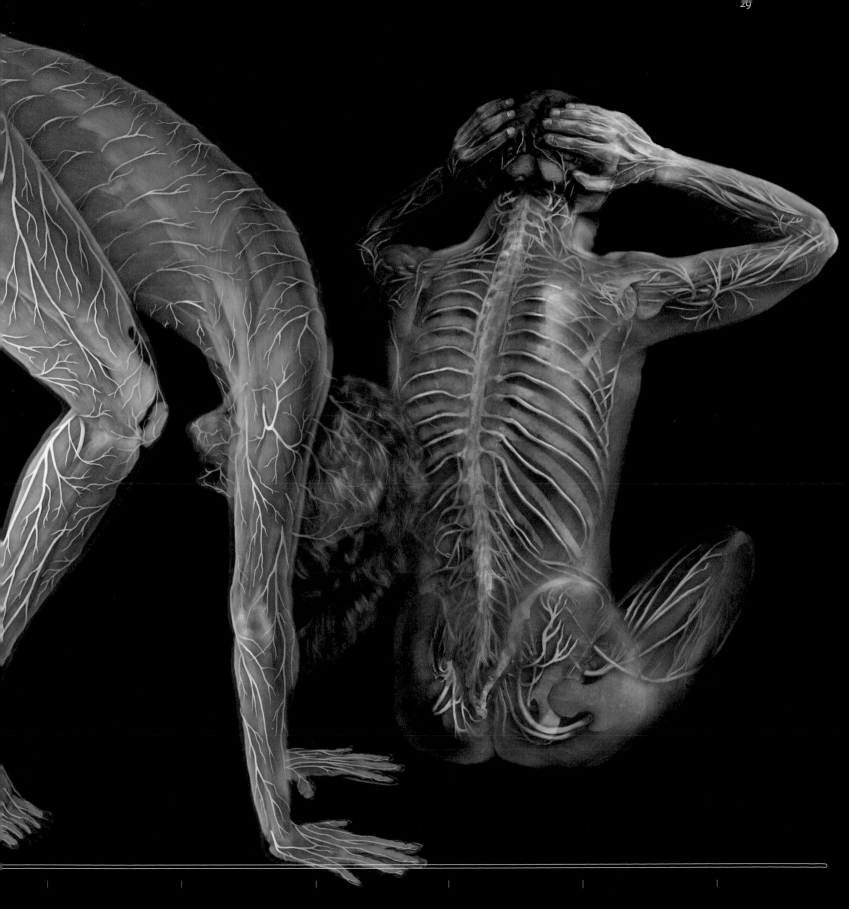

The universal dictum that nature builds from the bottom up is nowhere expressed more magnificently than in the development of the human brain. Barely 2 ½ weeks after conception, a spoonlike groove appears along the midline of the embryo's outermost layer of cells. At first, the cells running along the groove look no different than those around them, but as the groove deepens, then folds itself over into a cylinder, each new generation becomes progressively thinner, reeling out long filaments. Inside the tube, the rate of production of new cells—250,000 per minute—is staggering.

Within 10 days, the cells begin migrating, streaming over and past each other as if on invisible ladders. Complex and subtle chemical releases choreograph their movements as the nervous system, which eventually must carry signals to every cellular subsystem in the body, constructs itself literally from the inside out. New nerve channels weave themselves headlong into cables that ramify and connect over and over as the embryo becomes a fetus, and then, in the last trimester, undergoes explosive growth in the brain.

BUILDING THE GRID

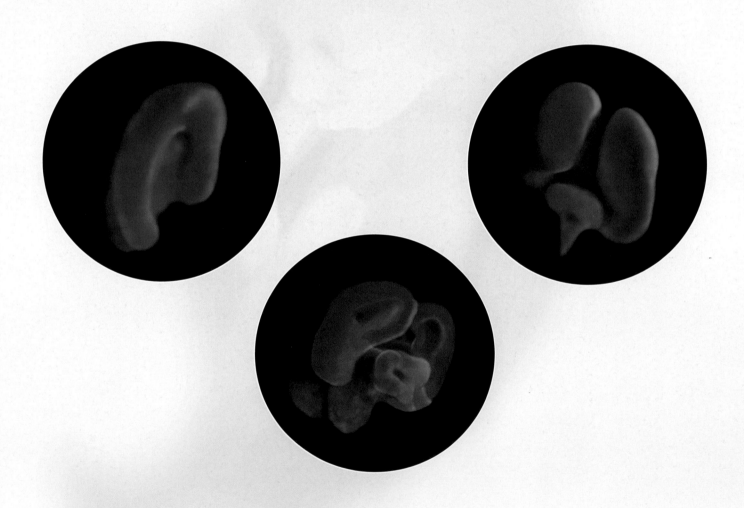

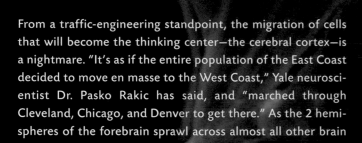

From a traffic-engineering standpoint, the migration of cells that will become the thinking center—the cerebral cortex—is a nightmare. "It's as if the entire population of the East Coast decided to move en masse to the West Coast," Yale neuroscientist Dr. Pasko Rakic has said, and "marched through Cleveland, Chicago, and Denver to get there." As the 2 hemispheres of the forebrain sprawl across almost all other brain structures in the seventh month, their surfaces erupt in precise folds—fissures—that in every normal human brain are located in precisely the same position, with identical depth, and with exactly the same connections to other fissures. The wiring map of this superstructure, which involves an estimated 10 trillion connections—some, in molecular terms, are thousands of miles long—would dwarf that of the Internet.

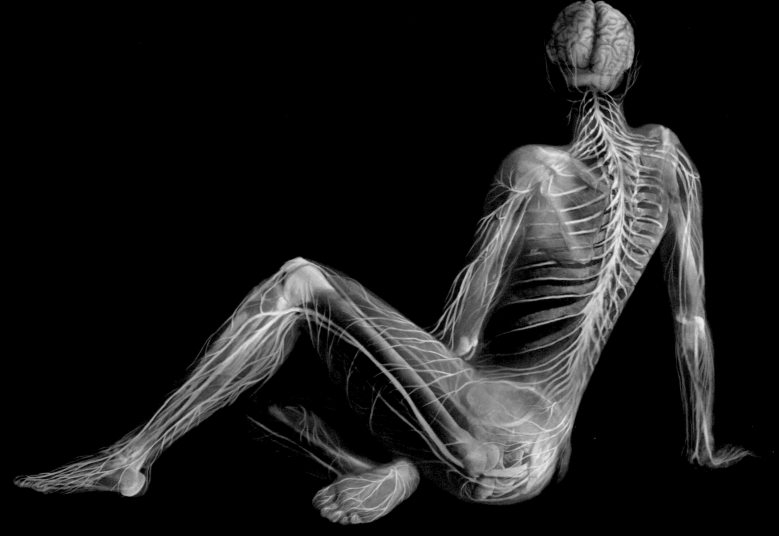

THE FULL SYSTEM

When the French master sculptor Auguste Rodin gave form to the suffering, malaise, and ennui of the nineteenth century in his famous creation "The Thinker," he celebrated a humanity virtually lost in deep thought. But it's the nonthinking portions of the nervous system that maintain control of the body, managing the multifaceted business of life so as to afford the upper brain the leisure to anguish over what it means.

Encased in the skull and spine, the tangles of nerves responsible for processing information and directing actions—the central nervous system (CNS)—are supremely capable but ultimately fragile: severed or injured, they don't grow back. By comparison, the 30,000 miles of nerves outside the CNS (the peripheral system) are individually less complex, yet they divide and branch to permeate as many body parts and tissues as possible and regrow lushly when harmed.

Attached along meridians extending the length and breadth of the body, the peripheral nerves are organized by function. Either they relay sensory information, stimulate voluntary muscles, or carry instructions to organs and glands. This last division is further cleaved into 2 distinct branches, the *sympathetic* or "fight or flight" branch, which in emergencies involuntarily makes you sweat as your heart pounds and your mouth gets dry, and the *parasympathetic*, which quiets the body and conserves energy when all is finally well.

GENDER DIFFERENCES

Fifty years ago, psychotherapist Carl Jung dismissed Freud's theory of sexuality as too mechanistic: "The brain," Jung spat, "is viewed as an appendage of the genital glands." In fact, researchers now understand that in men, the penis is under the complete control of the CNS, both during arousal and at rest, and that many regions of the brain contribute to male sexual response—from the hindbrain center that deepens breathing to areas in the cerebral cortex that concoct erotic fantasies. During arousal, excitatory signals either from the brain or from physical stimulation spur nerves in the penis to release chemicals that signal the smooth muscles of the arteries to relax and fill with blood, resulting in an erection. Switching off the activity

of the sympathetic nervous system also enhances erections, which explains why it's practically impossible to become sexually aroused while running from a bear.

In women, the sheer number of excitatory neurons makes for a more direct, unmediated sexual response. Consider the clitoris, which as writer Natalie Angier notes, "is simply a bundle of nerves; 8,000 nerve fibers, to be precise. That's a higher concentration of nerve fibers than is found anywhere else on the body, including the fingertips, lips, and tongue, and it is twice the number in the penis. In a sense, then, a woman's little brain is bigger than a man's." Touché, Dr. Freud.

MAN

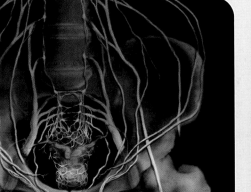

WOMAN

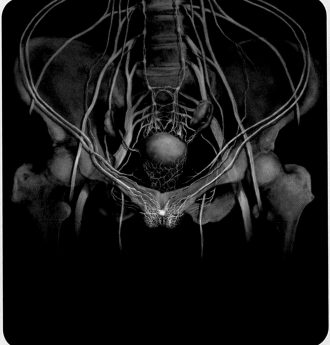

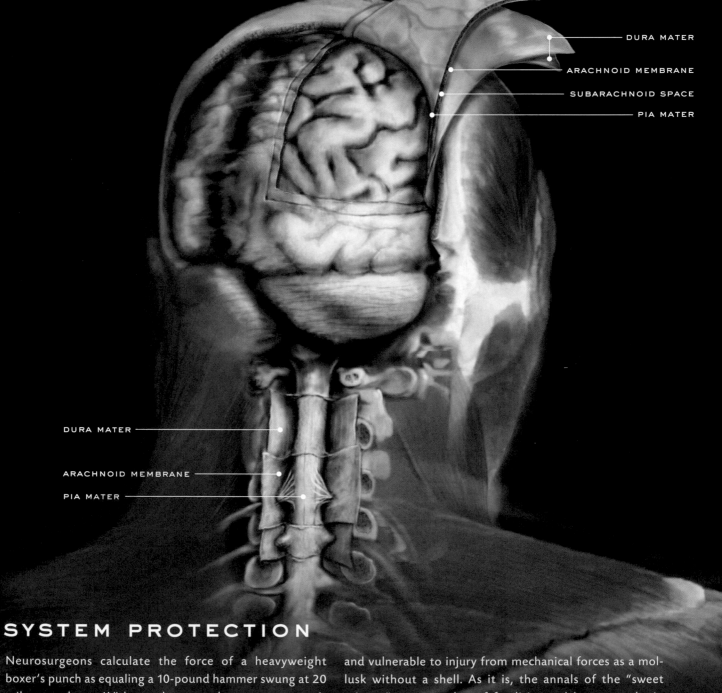

DURA MATER

ARACHNOID MEMBRANE

SUBARACHNOID SPACE

PIA MATER

DURA MATER

ARACHNOID MEMBRANE

PIA MATER

SYSTEM PROTECTION

Neurosurgeons calculate the force of a heavyweight boxer's punch as equaling a 10-pound hammer swung at 20 miles per hour. Without the central nervous system's extraordinary protective structures—an elaborate floatation system—our vital nerve centers would be as exposed and vulnerable to injury from mechanical forces as a mollusk without a shell. As it is, the annals of the "sweet science" are a catalog of fatalities and long-term brain damage from fighters taking repeated poundings to the head and neck.

A gently circulating liquid cushion separates the solid bones of the skull, which may fracture if struck hard enough, and the soft tissue of the brain; it also surrounds the spinal cord, where, massaged by the movements of the vertebrae, it sluices down along the back and up along the front of the cord. Like a soft laminate, 3 membranes—the meninges—cover the brain: an outermost coat, rich in blood vessels to nourish the skull; a middle layer of webbed, elastic connective tissue known as the arachnoid for its spidery texture; and conforming minutely to every fold, a delicate inner layer that contains the clear fluid.

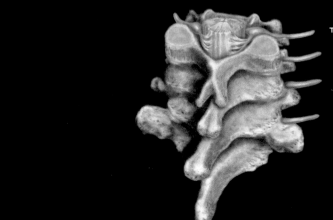

THE SPINAL CORD IS ENSCONCED WITH SPIKELIKE STRUCTURES TETHERING THE SYSTEM TO THE VERTEBRAE.

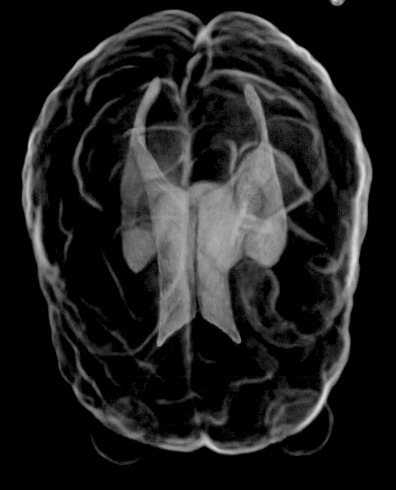

HORN-SHAPED CHAMBERS UNDER THE CEREBRUM PRODUCE AND RELEASE THE FLUID THROUGH A MAIN AQUEDUCT INTO THIS CEREBROSPINAL FLUID SYSTEM, LIKE A PUMPHOUSE LODGED AT THE CENTER OF WATERWORKS. HOWEVER, SINCE THE CHAMBERS HAVE NO MECHANICAL CAPACITY THEMSELVES, CIRCULATION IS HELPED ALONG BY THE PULSING OF NEARBY BLOOD VESSELS.

Sight and hearing had passed into her hands—hands that create light out of darkness, sound out of perpetual silence, and alone bring her into communion with nature and her own kind.
—Photographer Yousef Karsh on his portrait of Helen Keller, which focuses equally on Keller's hands and face

When God reaches out to Adam in Michelangelo's classic rendering of Creation, it is with a "mighty" right hand. But hands are also multipronged antennae equipped for exquisite dexterity, designed to send and receive the most delicate messages—to touch. Long before a newborn's eyes can focus

SENSE AND MOTION

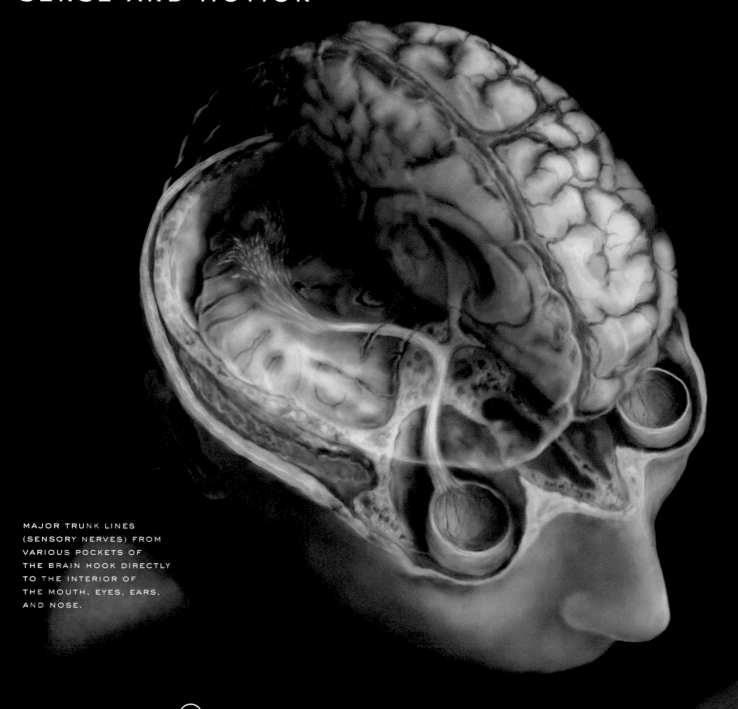

MAJOR TRUNK LINES
(SENSORY NERVES) FROM
VARIOUS POCKETS OF
THE BRAIN HOOK DIRECTLY
TO THE INTERIOR OF
THE MOUTH, EYES, EARS,
AND NOSE.

on an object or the sounds that she hears become intelligible to her, the skin on her palms and fingers, filigreed with neurons, is her chief instrument for discerning the world. Two distinct nerve groups are at work—those that send motor signals to the dozens of muscles that flex and release, together and separately, the hand's 27 bones, which distribute the force of movement; and those that supply the skin. On the inside of the hand, these latter consist of 2 branching groups that subdivide in the palm, then bow, like tweezers, until they reach the tips of the fingers, where touch is most sensitive.

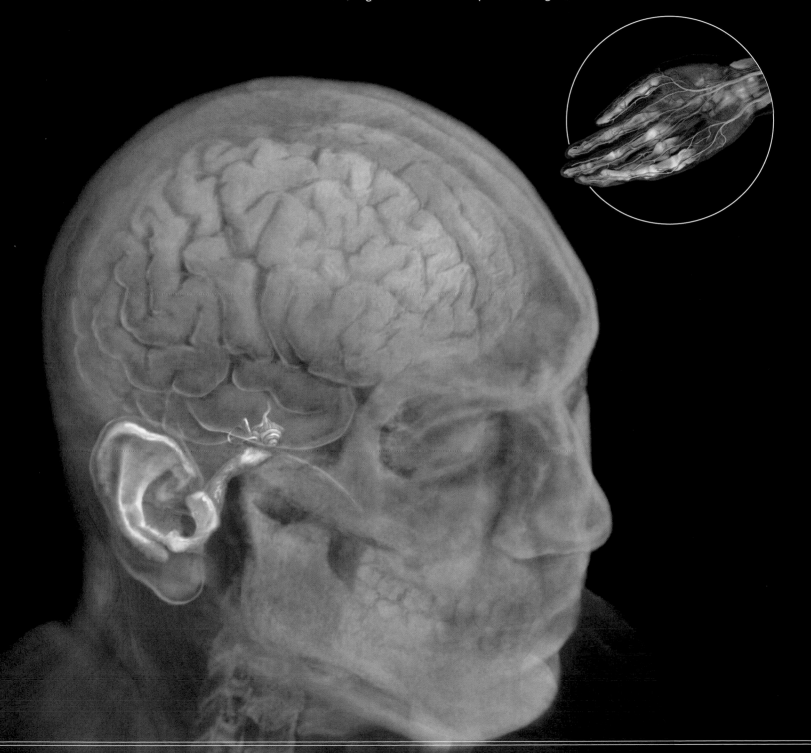

During the forties at MIT, the visionary mathematician Norbert Weiner combined advances in computers and wartime research into the nervous system to create a new field—cybernetics—which he defined as "control and communication in the animal and the machine." Weiner's father was acquainted with the physiologist Walter Cannon, who a decade earlier had observed that the human body, like other complex systems ranging from cells to global corporations, maintains a certain inner balance. Weiner identified the central mechanism involved in keeping this inner balance as the *feedback* loop—a series of structures that carry a circular cascade of information. Like D'Arcy and Turing, he believed that biological mechanisms could be understood through engineering and math, and cybernetics now influences much modern thinking about systems, from how molecules communicate within cells, to economics, to how to guide rockets and manage the growth of the Internet.

FEEDBACK LOOPS

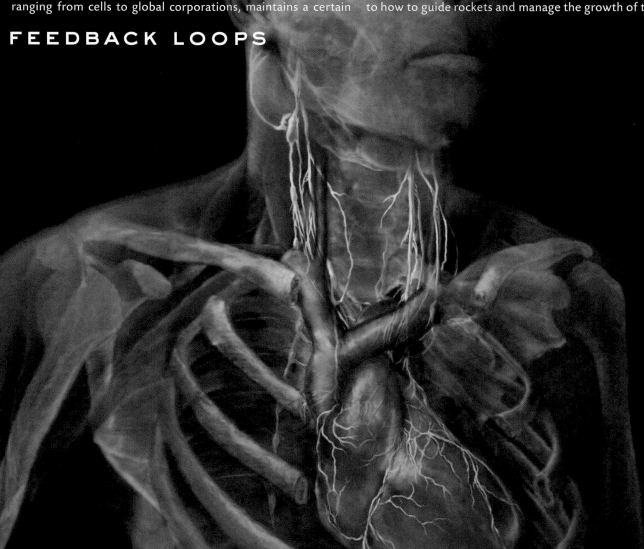

Crowning the neural feedback system in humans is the hypothalamus, a fingernail-sized, funnel-shaped, downward-pointing cluster of discrete tissues in the midbrain. The joke about this "King of Glands"—which automatically controls not only breathing, appetite, thirst, and heart rate but also the hormones governing digestion, body chemistry, and sex—is that it maintains and balances the four F's of survival: fight, flight, feeding, and mating. With direct neural connections to the cardiovascular (ABOVE) and digestive complexes (RIGHT), and with master control over the endocrine system, the hypothalamus is a feedback virtuoso.

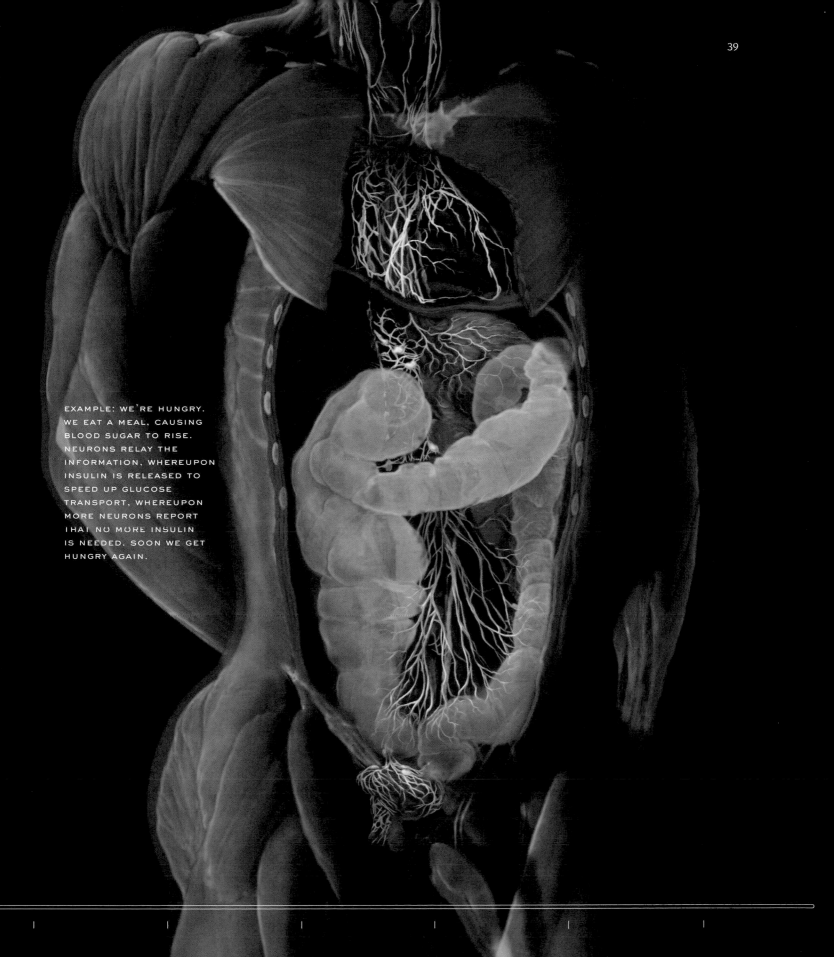

EXAMPLE: WE'RE HUNGRY.
WE EAT A MEAL, CAUSING
BLOOD SUGAR TO RISE.
NEURONS RELAY THE
INFORMATION, WHEREUPON
INSULIN IS RELEASED TO
SPEED UP GLUCOSE
TRANSPORT, WHEREUPON
MORE NEURONS REPORT
THAT NO MORE INSULIN
IS NEEDED. SOON WE GET
HUNGRY AGAIN.

During the first half of the nineteenth century, it was widely believed that by examining the topography of the skull—its bumps and depressions—one could "read" the intellectual aptitudes and character traits of a human mind. Phrenology, as it was called ("bumpology" to its detractors), stemmed from the notion that every mental faculty has a specific location on the surface of the brain. Since the size of a locale was thought to be a measure of its power, and since the skull takes its shape from the brain, phrenologists believed they could employ fingers and calipers to explore a person's personality. At the height of the phrenology craze, before the practice was hijacked by racial supremacists and others seeking a simple, physiological index of intelligence, employers could demand a character reference from a local phrenologist, just as many corporations today demand urine tests to measure a worker's reliability.

Though skull mapping was a crude, socially dangerous methodology, phrenology's basic premise—localizing the functions of thought and behavior among the outer contours of the cerebrum—has largely been vindicated by research. The cerebral hemispheres are covered with a thin, folded grayish sheet of nerve cell bodies called the cortex, which ranges in thickness from $1/8$ to $1/5$ inch—about the width of a pencil. This is the seat of all thinking, with different types of neurons distributed differently across the 6 layers of this "gray

SHEER INTELLIGENCE

BRAIN AND NERVOUS SYSTEM

THALAMUS

HYPOTHALAMUS

HIPPOCAMPUS

LEFT CEREBRAL
HEMISPHERE

PONS

CEREBELLUM

MEDULLA OBLONGATA

SPINAL CORD

2

matter," and different areas producing different functions. Unsurprisingly, the size of a cluster *does* matter. Studies indicate that professional musicians, for instance, have more gray matter than nonmusicians in the part of the brain that makes sense of sound tones. Using MRI and other scanning techniques, neurologists now superimpose knowledge of the brain's architecture onto what's known about how individuals function, to try to understand why they think and act as they do—the same mysteries Victorian phrenologists tried to divine.

The most significant epoch in brain development occurs during the first year or two *after* birth, when the brain's higher centers explode with not new cells but new *synapses*—those junction points between neurons where an impulse traveling as electricity in one, leaps, via a lightning-fast sequence of chemical reactions, to initiate an impulse in another. The number of synapses in a single layer of the brain's vision center rises from about 2,500 per neuron at birth to as many as 18,000 at 6 months, as the infant first learns to see, then to discern distances. Similarly spectacular increases occur throughout the cortex as the newborn also learns to hear, smell, respond, touch, reach, grab, and soon, speak. This discovery has led most researchers to conclude that the chief architect of the brain after birth is not what's encoded in our genes but the experience of learning itself—that is, nurture over nature.

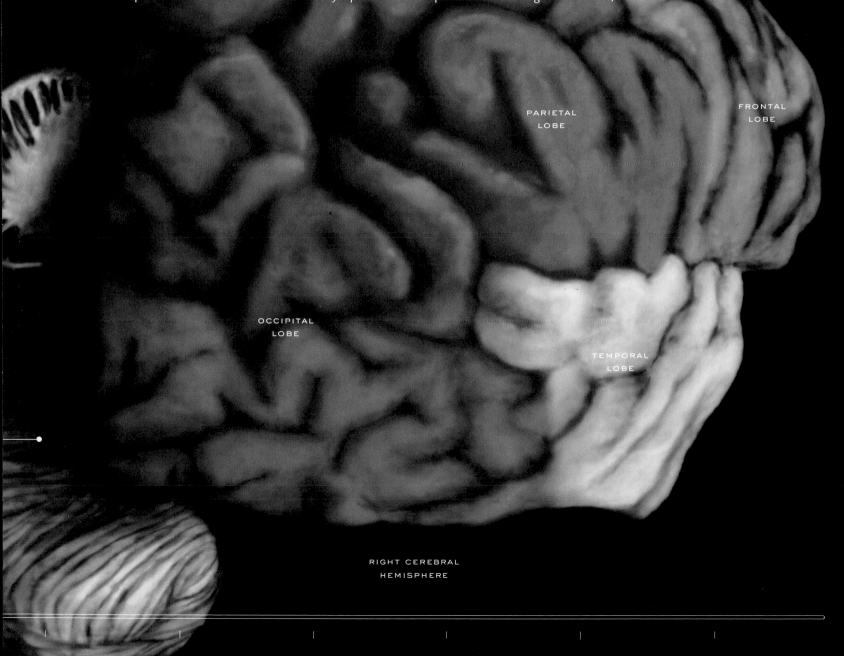

PARIETAL
LOBE

FRONTAL
LOBE

OCCIPITAL
LOBE

TEMPORAL
LOBE

RIGHT CEREBRAL
HEMISPHERE

The neurologist Paul MacLean has suggested that our skulls hold not 1 brain but 3, and that each stratum represents an evolutionary advance over an older sublayer, as in an archaeological dig. Imagine an office building built atop a medieval fort built atop an ancient temple. Yet in MacLean's analogy, the lower realms aren't merely vestigial ruins; they function, but primitively. All 3 edifices are connected, yet operate independent of one another, each "with its own special intelligence, its own subjectivity, its own sense of time and space, and its own memory." This counters the traditional hierarchical view of the mind, which holds that the highest level (rational thinking) dominates the brain's other functions, and MacLean has shown that the lower systems can override higher mental functions when necessary.

CORE FORMS

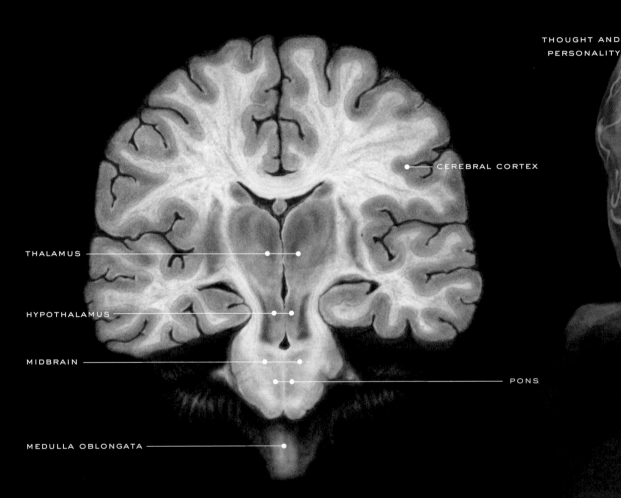

THOUGHT AND PERSONALITY

CEREBRAL CORTEX

THALAMUS

HYPOTHALAMUS

MIDBRAIN

PONS

MEDULLA OBLONGATA

BRAIN AND NERVOUS SYSTEM

Lofted above it is a walnut sized, ring-like series of structures comprising the "intermediate" brain, which is concerned with feelings and instincts. Power-packed with functions, this region sets a person's emotional tone, "tagging" memories and events with a valence, or charge, so that we know how to act. In addition, a pair of direct connections to bulb-shaped receptors in the nose help explain why certain smells evoke long-forgotten memories and emotions. Do we approach or pull back? Love or hate? The surrounding cerebral cortex—the office tower—may be responsible for problem solving, planning, and organization, but this fortified inner region, which registers and stores emotional memories, dictates how we *feel* about our experience.

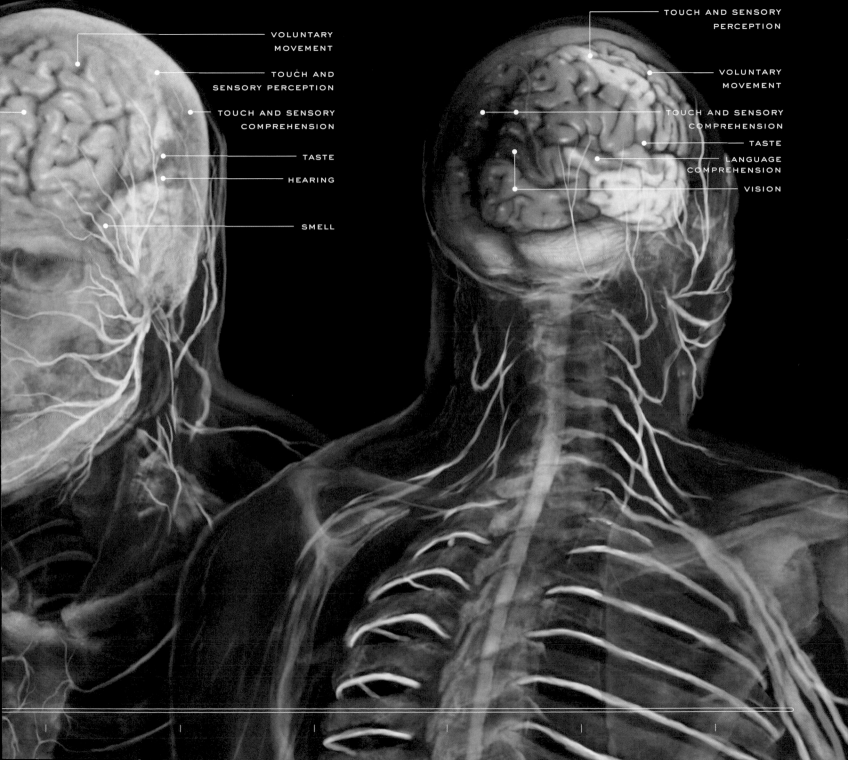

VOLUNTARY MOVEMENT

TOUCH AND SENSORY PERCEPTION

TOUCH AND SENSORY COMPREHENSION

TASTE

HEARING

SMELL

TOUCH AND SENSORY PERCEPTION

VOLUNTARY MOVEMENT

TOUCH AND SENSORY COMPREHENSION

TASTE

LANGUAGE COMPREHENSION

VISION

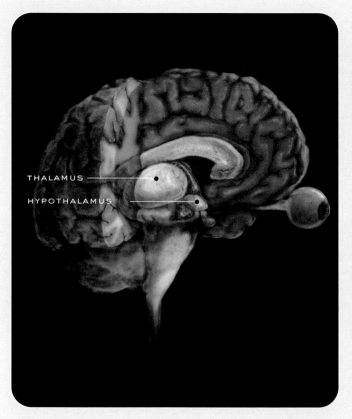

THALAMUS

HYPOTHALAMUS

MAN

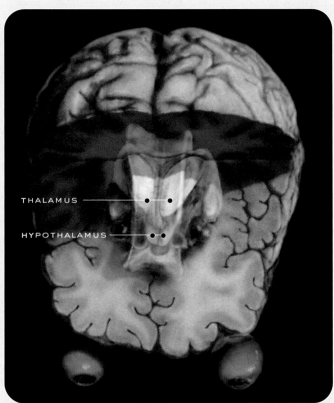

THALAMUS

HYPOTHALAMUS

WOMAN

DIFFERENCES BETWEEN MEN AND WOMEN

Neurobiologists have reported structural differences in 2 primary areas of the human brain: the main connecting cable between the hemispheres, and the hypothalamus, center of the primitive brain's feedback system. A cell cluster in the front part of the hypothalamus, thought to help direct sexual behavior, is twice as large in men, with double the number of neurons. Meanwhile, another cluster that acts as a built-in clock—governing circadian rhythms and, in women, ovulation—has a more elongated shape in females, although scientists have yet to determine any corresponding functional distinction.

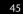

RIGHT CEREBRAL
HEMISPHERE

HYPOTHALAMUS

HIPPOCAMPUS

PITUITARY GLAND

MIDBRAIN

PONS

BRAIN STEM

MEDULLA OBLONGATA

The oldest brain—the ancient temple, so to speak—consists of
the conical structures of the brain stem. Active even in deep
sleep, this archaic center controls muscles, balance, breathing,
and heart rate, and is often called the "reptilian brain"
because, as in snakes and lizards, its behavioral program is
obsessive, ritualistic, and paranoid. It governs the most rudi-
mentary elements of survival.

Fanning out in pairs like the axes on a sundial, 12 skeins of nerve fibers—in some cases, a million or more—sprout from the undersurface of the brain, most relating to activities in the head and neck. Each pair coordinates a specific sensory and/or motor activity, connecting at the far end either with muscle cells, glands, or organs; or else with specialized nerve clusters, such as taste buds and light receptors in the eye, that glean information from the outside world.

ROTARY DIAL

I   OLFACTORY NERVE—connects with the inside of the nose; relays information about smells

II   OPTIC NERVE—a bundle of about a million fibers; sends visual signals from the retina to the brain

III   (IV, VI) OCULOMOTOR, TROCHLEAR, ABDUCENS NERVES—carry stimuli for voluntary movements of the eye muscles and eyelids; control pupil dilation and lens changes during focusing

IV   SEE III

V   TRIGEMINAL NERVE—branches into 3 bundles: relays signals from the head, face, and teeth; innervates muscles involved in chewing

VI   SEE III

VII   FACIAL NERVE—ramifies to connect with taste buds, skin of the outer ear, salivary glands, and tear glands; also controls facial expressions

VIII   VESTIBULOCOCHLEAR NERVE—sensory fibers transmit information about sound balance from the inner ear to the brain

IX   GLOSSOPHARYNGEAL—motor fibers control swallowing while sensory fibers transmit information from the tongue and pharynx about pain, taste, touch, and heat

X   VAGUS NERVE—meaning "wanderer," these fibers connect to many muscles, glands, and organs, including the heart, lungs, and stomach; involved innumerous involuntary functions, including digestion and heartbeat

XI   ACCESSORY NERVE—controls movement of muscles involved in swallowing, moving the head, and producing voice sounds

XII   HYPOGLOSSAL NERVE—meaning "under the tongue," these nerves control many of the muscles in the tongue associated with speech

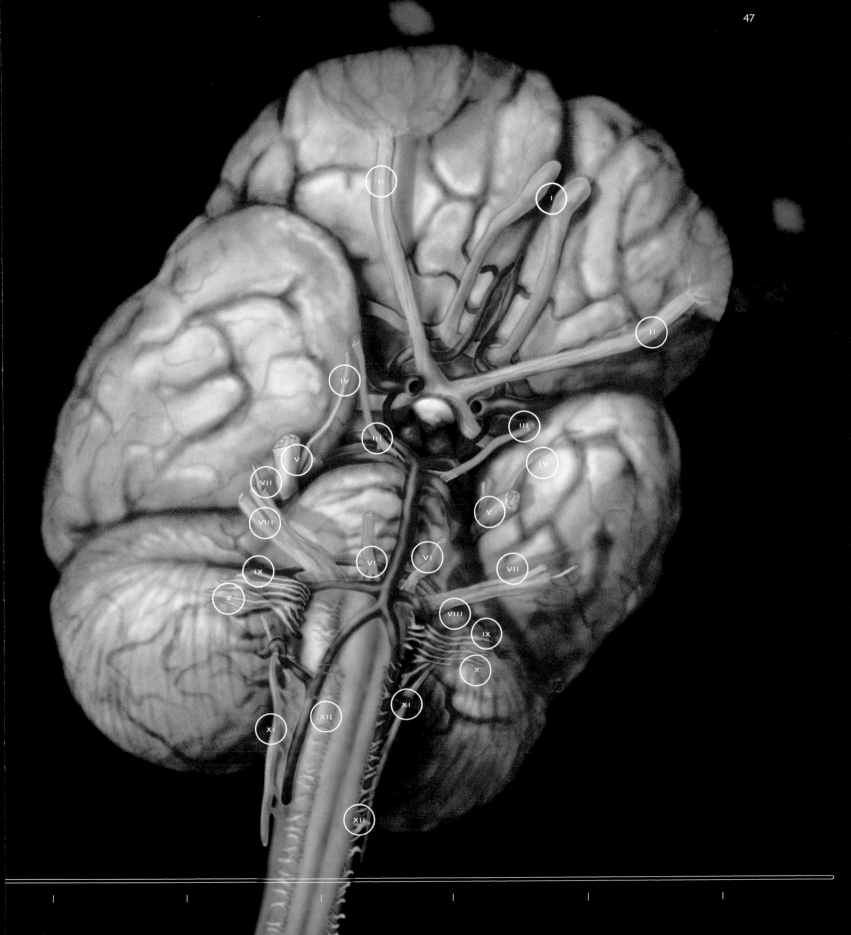

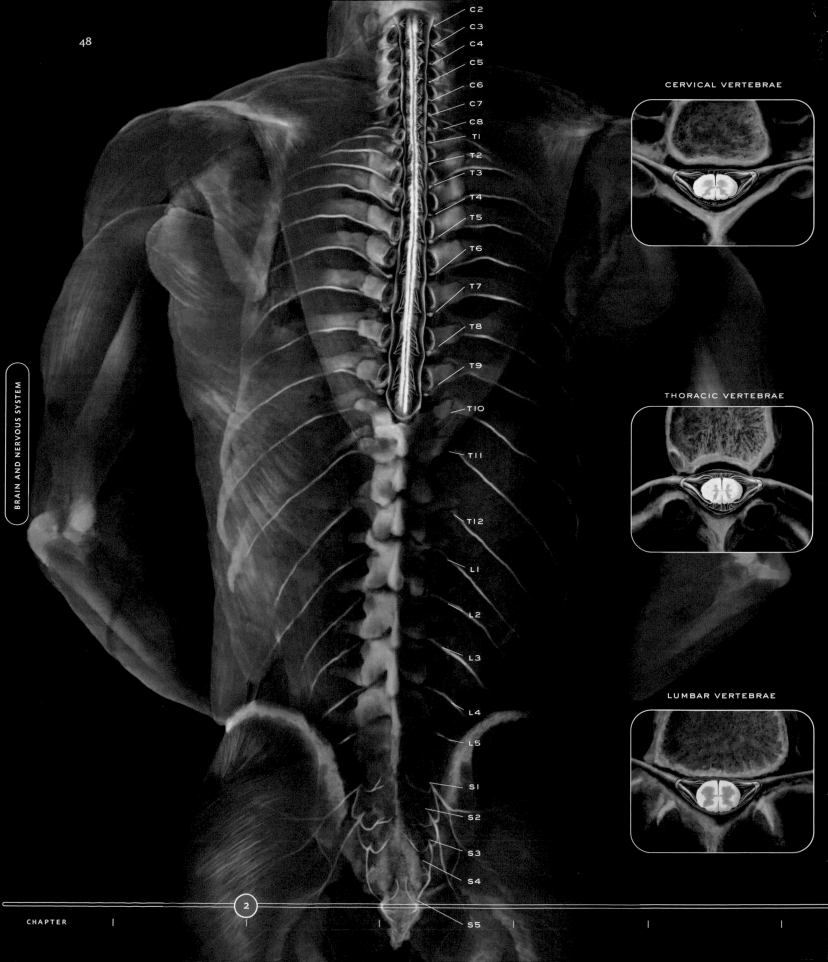

C2
C3
C4
C5
C6
C7
C8
T1
T2
T3
T4
T5
T6
T7
T8
T9
T10
T11
T12
L1
L2
L3
L4
L5
S1
S2
S3
S4
S5

CERVICAL VERTEBRAE

THORACIC VERTEBRAE

LUMBAR VERTEBRAE

BRAIN AND NERVOUS SYSTEM

Like any other towering corporate entity, the body requires rapid, 2-way communications with all its territories. Branching symmetrically from the spinal cord, 29 pairs of cables penetrate every inch of muscle and skin and every gland, via a 30,000-mile network that relays information almost instantaneously to and from the brain.

SITE MAP

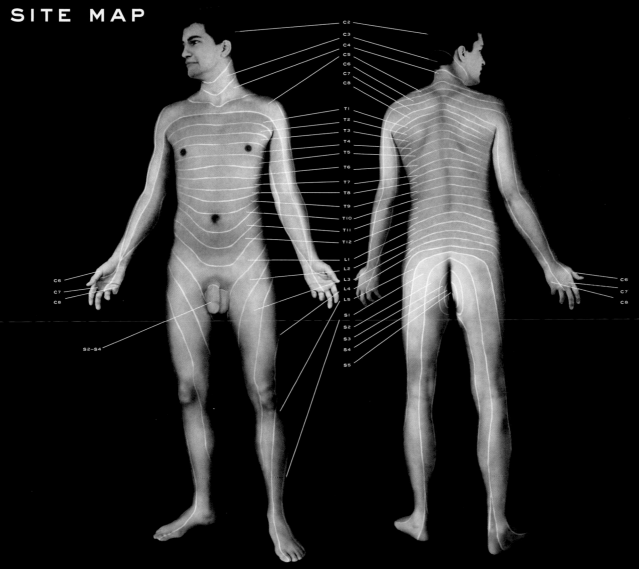

Fortunately for us, the organizational chart for this network—which allows doctors to identify and fix problems within the system—is tattooed invisibly on our skin. The peripheral nerves—the main trunk lines—subdivide the body into front and back, then again by region. The regions in the trunk are roughly horizontal, but those in the limbs are aligned lengthwise. By mapping the skin with needle pricks, neurologists divide the body into zones, called dermatomes, which enable them to track backward into the peripheral nervous system in order to locate injured areas. However, since the zones overlap slightly, nerve distribution can only be approximated.

Sometimes branches from different spinal nerves intertwine and become braided in order to serve areas of complex function and movement, such as the shoulder and neck. These braids, called plexuses, have lately become a common metaphor in industries like software, computer graphics, and Web design and development, where a key architectural challenge is to create mechanisms that mesh and overlap with other systems.

Nerves are bundles of live wires. The basic unit—though much more than just a wire itself—is the gangly, whiplike structure of the *neuron*.

Like other cells, neurons are designed to interact with each other. But the nature, volume, variety, and some of the distances involved in these interactions require a specialized, hydra-headed design—like an octopus with 2 types of tendrils.

REAL LIVE WIRES

Firing in collective bursts, neurons are designed to send and receive electrical messages—flashes—along a number of filaments. The longest of these extensions (some reach up to 3 feet) carry messages away from the cell body, and are called *axons*. To help speed up transmission, axons are padded with packets of fatty insulation, then bundled into gangs, wrapped, and rebundled into cables that can relay a flash at speeds over 200 miles per hour. A single neuron can have 100 connections. In other words, instant group messaging.

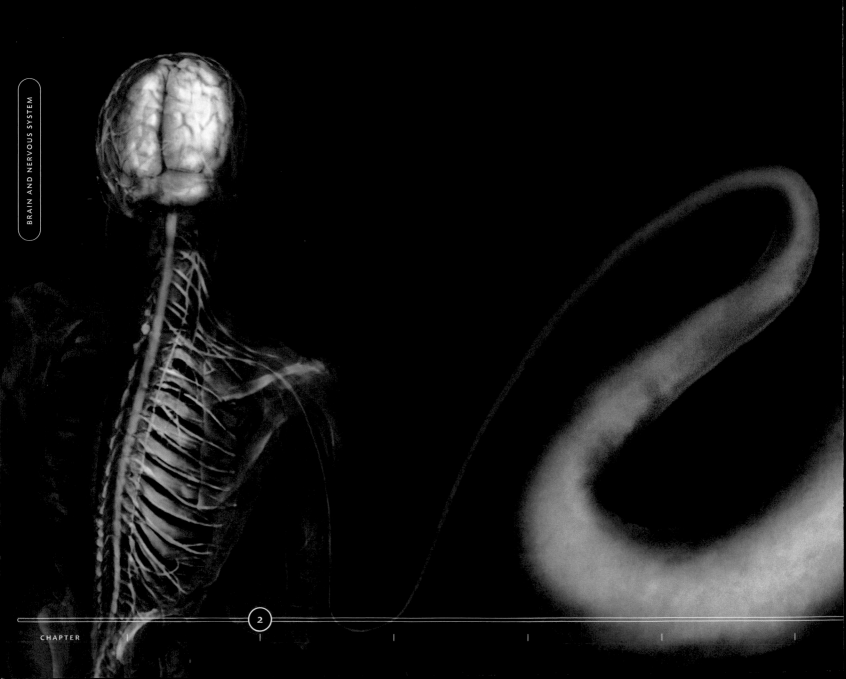

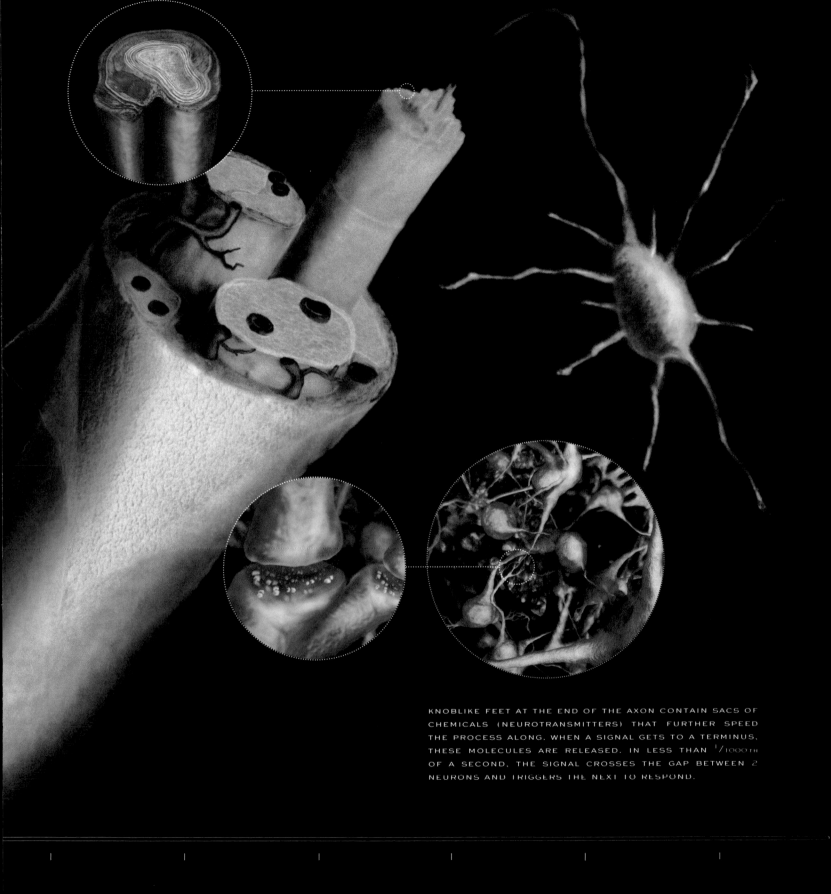

KNOBLIKE FEET AT THE END OF THE AXON CONTAIN SACS OF CHEMICALS (NEUROTRANSMITTERS) THAT FURTHER SPEED THE PROCESS ALONG. WHEN A SIGNAL GETS TO A TERMINUS, THESE MOLECULES ARE RELEASED. IN LESS THAN $^1/_{1000\text{TH}}$ OF A SECOND, THE SIGNAL CROSSES THE GAP BETWEEN 2 NEURONS AND TRIGGERS THE NEXT TO RESPOND.

MIRRORED IN NATURE

The kinship we sense, and beauty we perceive, in nature often reflect deep structural connections between what's us and what's not—"transcendental geometry," the poet and philosopher Paul Valéry called it. Cross-sectioned, the spinal cord resembles nothing so much as a butterfly, a floor plan of fissures and columns. Thrust-out extensions—horns—of white and gray matter are shaped like greater and lesser wings. The climbing, mossy circuitry of the cerebellum has a framework similar to certain

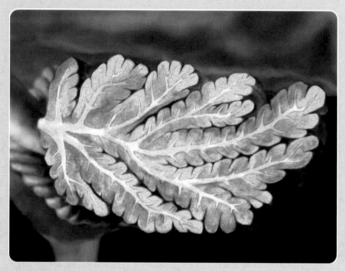

CEREBELLUM

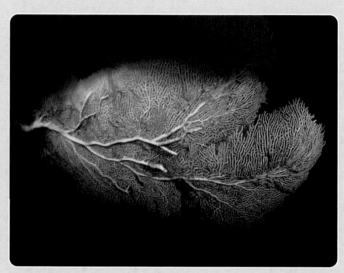

SALT WATER CORAL

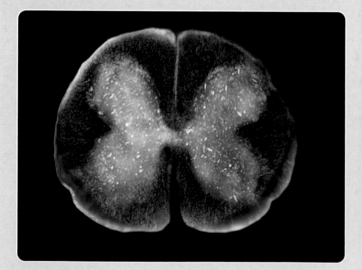

SPINAL CORD

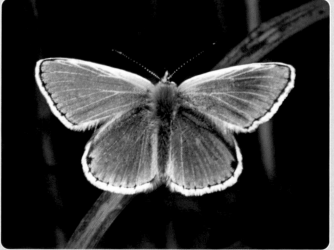

BUTTERFLY

filigreed sea corals, while brain corals, their brawnier cousins, have dense channels and grooves on their surfaces that look like the folds of the human brain. (It's hard to argue the relative intelligence of reef creatures, but brain corals hold their ground by being solid and strong enough to withstand storms that pound more delicate corals to rubble.)

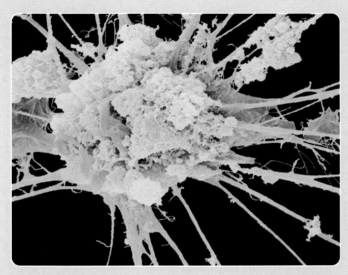

NERVOUS TISSUE

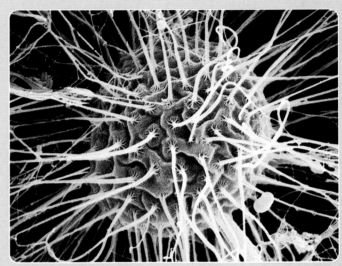

GREEN ALGA

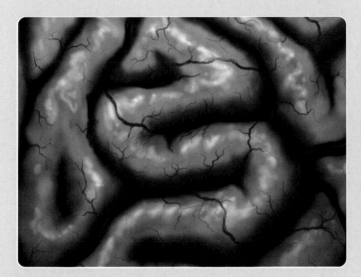

CEREBRAL CORTEX

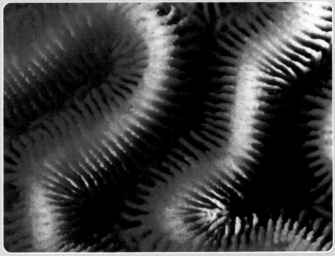

FOLDS OF BRAIN CORAL

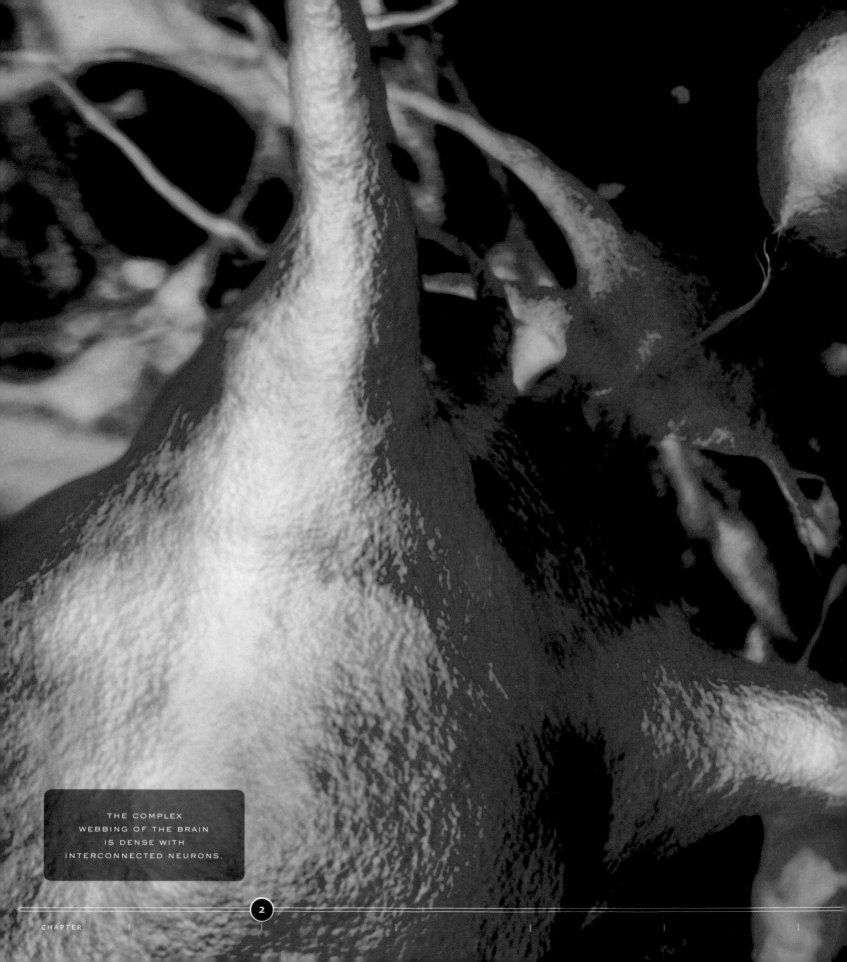

THE COMPLEX
WEBBING OF THE BRAIN
IS DENSE WITH
INTERCONNECTED NEURONS.

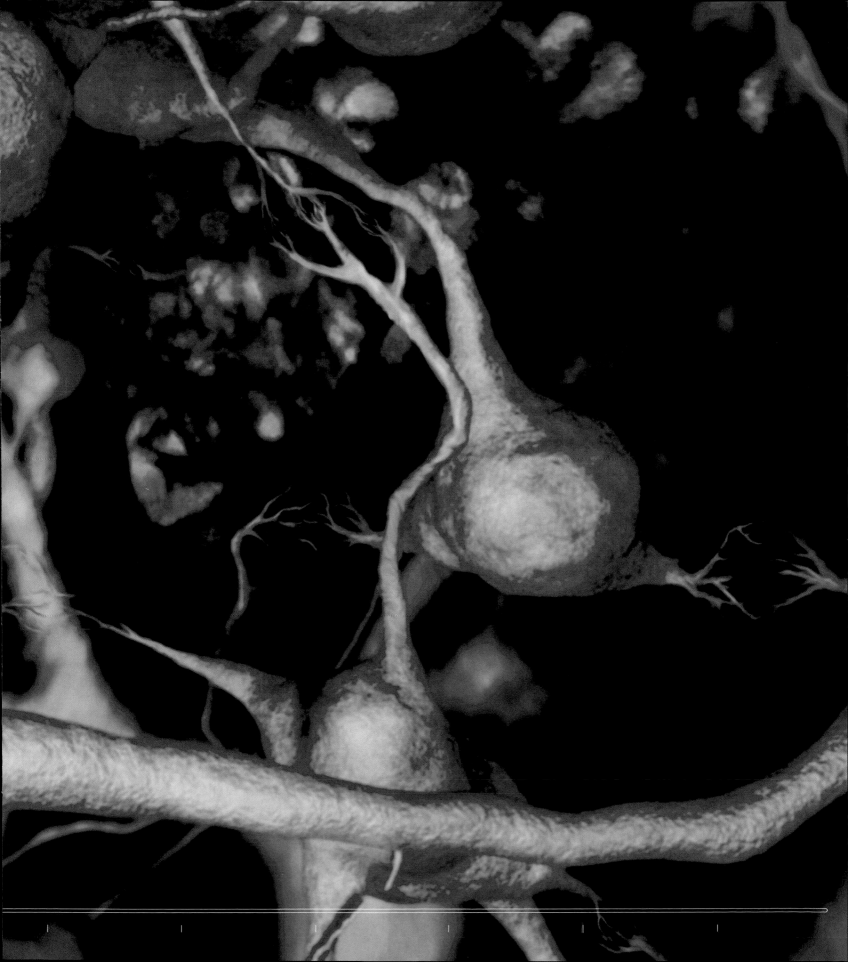

sensory

(senses)

Lovers close their eyes when they kiss because, if they didn't, there would be too many visual distractions to notice and analyze—the sudden close-up of the loved one's eyelashes and hair, the wallpaper, the clock face, the dust motes suspended in a shaft of sunlight. Lovers want to do serious touching, and not be disturbed. So they close their eyes as if asking two cherished relatives to leave the room.
—Diane Ackerman, *A Natural History of the Senses*

Portals to the outside world, the contact senses are specialized extensions of the central nervous system designed to gather and relay information. The smell of a baby's scalp, the sight of a hawk, the taste of a lover's lips, a needle prick: all involve sub-microscopic receptors receiving stimuli at very localized sites and passing electrochemical signals along a high-speed network, evoking a response. Biologically speaking, Ackerman is right: in order to focus, we can only take in and process so much sensory information at one time.

The data we receive is another matter, since in it lies the *experience* of life. Everything we see, hear, smell, taste, and feel forms our knowledge of the world and of ourselves, triggering cascades of association and emotion. "We are all instruments endowed with feeling and memory," the French philosopher Denis Diderot wrote, in 1769. "Our senses are so many strings that are struck by surrounding objects and that also frequently strike themselves."

CONTACT ZONE

Beauty through my senses stole;
I yielded myself to the perfect whole.
—Ralph Waldo Emerson

Enveloping the body like a force field, our contact senses connect us to the world, especially to each other. A pregnant woman, her estrogen rising, abruptly smells and tastes foods more keenly, perhaps as a protective mechanism for herself and her child. At birth, the newborn is overloaded with sensory input but quickly learns, starting with a breast, to put everything in her mouth so as to absorb life through her lips and tongue, which along with fingertips have the highest density of touch receptors in the body. Babies find comfort and safety in familiar (albeit unintelligible) voices, as they learn to use their eyes in tandem to differentiate among objects and people. By age 6 or 7—the Catholic Age of Reason, when moral responsibility starts—the sensory apparatus is fully developed and integrated, and at the peak of our youth our eyes and ears detect wider ranges of light and sound than they will in adulthood.

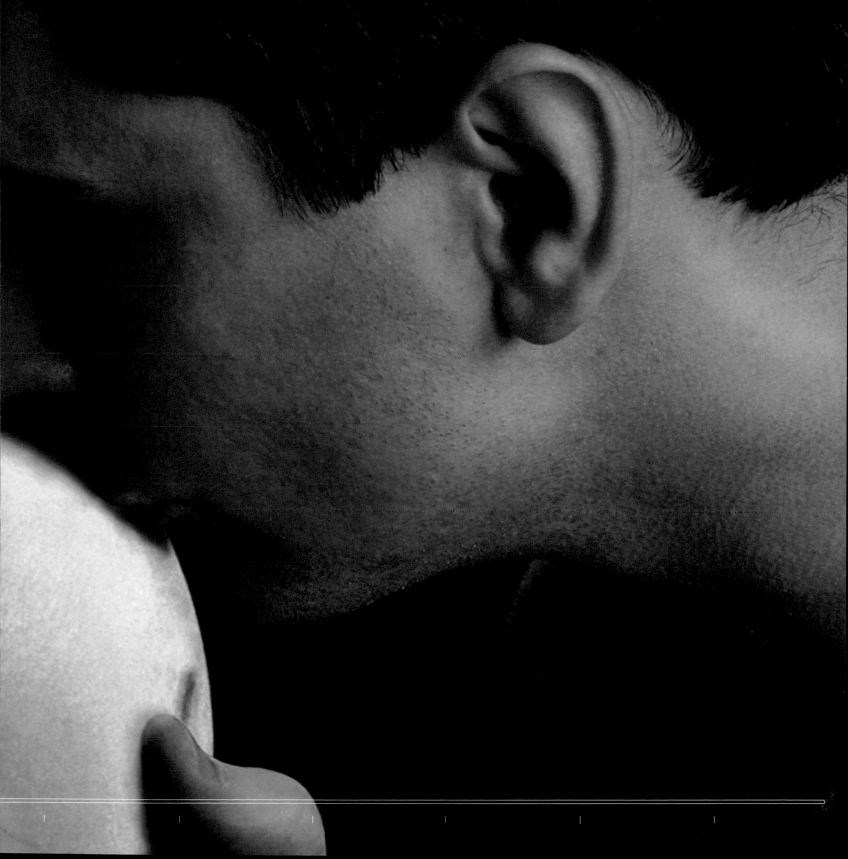

What our sensory detectors pick up out of the atmosphere and from contact with our own bodies is vast, yet almost nothing compared with what's out there. There are toxic particles in the air we can't smell, sound frequencies too high or too low for us (but not other animals) to hear, ribbons of the rainbow we can't see. It is the range of stimuli a sense organ is attuned to—and its connection to a specific region of the brain—that establishes its functional design: its structures, what they're made of, how the parts assemble and connect.

Like other scanning devices, biological sensors need energy to function: the more receptor cells in an area, the higher the blood requirement, and the more developed the

arterial design. The sensitivity of the fingertips, so acute that blind people can read by touch, is accomplished in part by oxygenated blood flooding into the nail bed through a complex network of arteries that shadows the branching nerves. The nose has a dual blood supply, which explains why nosebleeds can be stanched by applying pressure to the upper front gum. High blood flow to the tongue helps account for its redness and the fact that, when cut, it heals faster than other parts of the body. The convergence of blood vessels and nerves at a common exit point on the back of the eyeball creates a disk-shaped "blind spot" on the retina that has no photoreceptors and thus can't detect light.

SENSITIVITY

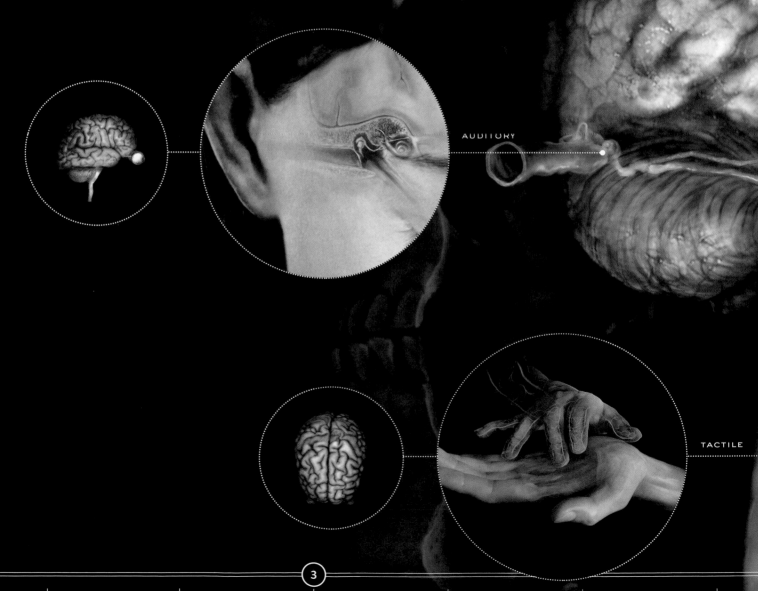

AUDITORY

TACTILE

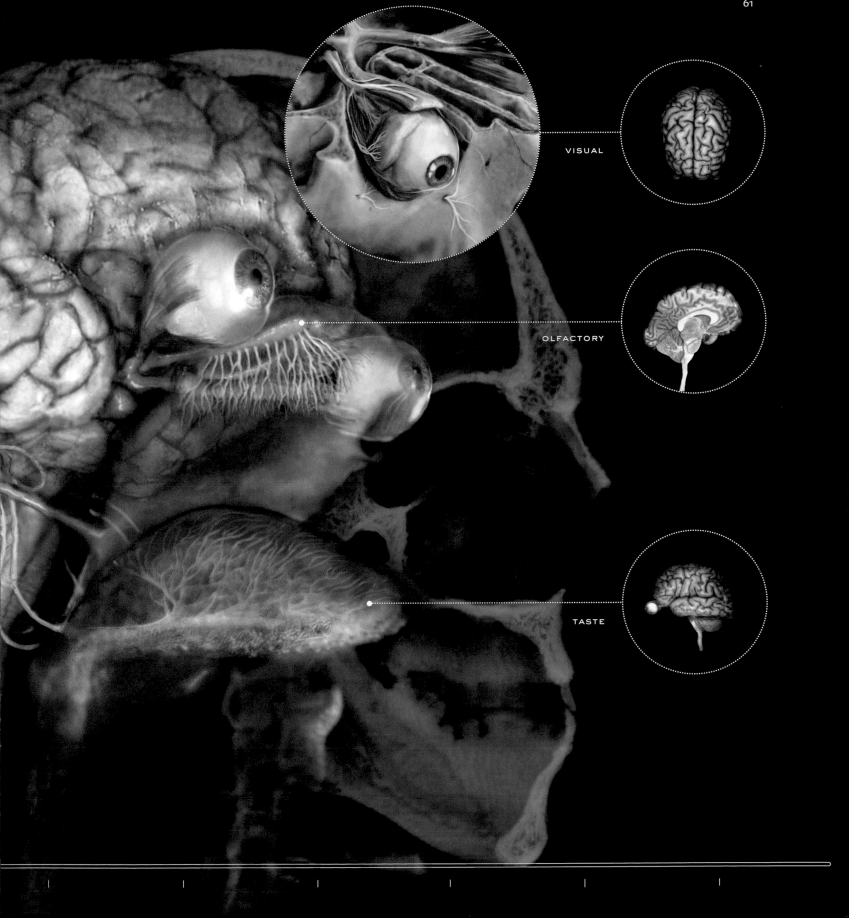

VISUAL

OLFACTORY

TASTE

THE HUMAN TOUCH

With more sensory receptors than any other organ, the skin is a full-body scanning network, a continental radar system able to register movements as traumatic as a burn and as minor as individual hairs rustled by a breeze. Each receptor is a listening device, its structure and mechanics determined by what type of information is being listened for, and how near it is to the surface. Disklike cells (A) imbedded in the epidermis sense slight changes in touch and pressure, and help pinpoint the source. The last branches of nerve axons intertwine with basketlike arrays of cells in the dermis below to form microphonelike probes (D), also aimed at the surface. Deeper, spraylike corpuscles (B) sense steady pressure, and beyond

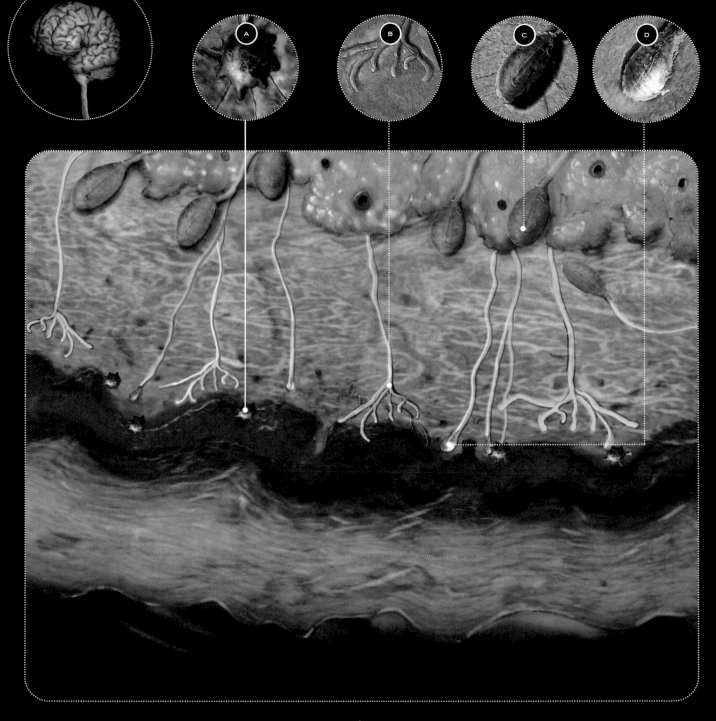

those are still more encapsulated receptors (c), larger and flatter, which respond to vibration and strong pressure deep inside the skin. Together, they signal a strip on the brain's surface, the somatosensory cortex, or touch center.

In the 1930s, Canadian brain surgeon Wilder Penfield mapped the touch network by stimulating this area to see what regions of the skin were affected. To illustrate his findings, Penfield invented a cartoon character, a *homunculus* (little man), drawing its features according to how much brain space they take up. Lips, tongues, fingers, toes, and footsoles, with their vastly greater numbers of receptors, are larger than arms and legs.

a near one, the rubbery, convex lens of the eye works the way a camera does, adjusting the distance between the opening and the chemical surface. Clustered at the back of the eyeball—a kind of biological movie screen where light converges and images form—are specialized nerve cells, each packed with up to 100 million molecules of light-sensitive pigment that convert light into electrochemical signals. When a smaller molecule (retinal) within the pigment receives light energy in the form of a "packet," it twists its backbone, launching a chain of chemical reactions.

LIGHTS, ACTION

Though the great majority of the retinal cells—about 100 million—are *rods*, which work best in dim light but cannot distinguish color, several million *cones* conduct color, but only respond to bright light. Because genes for the red and green color receptors are located on the female sex chromosome, genetic red-green colorblindness affects men much more often than women. The difference is purely mathematical: women are red-green colorblind if both their X chromosomes are affected; men if their only X chromosome is defective, which means that the incidence in males is the square of that in females. (In the United States, about 8 percent of men and 0.5 percent of women have some difficulty discerning colors.)

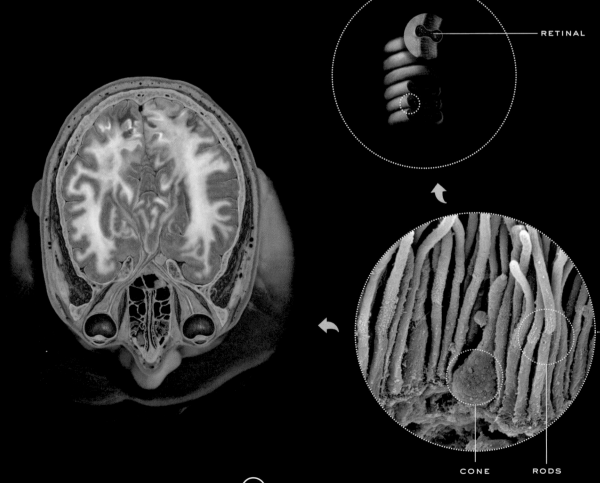

RETINAL

CONE   RODS

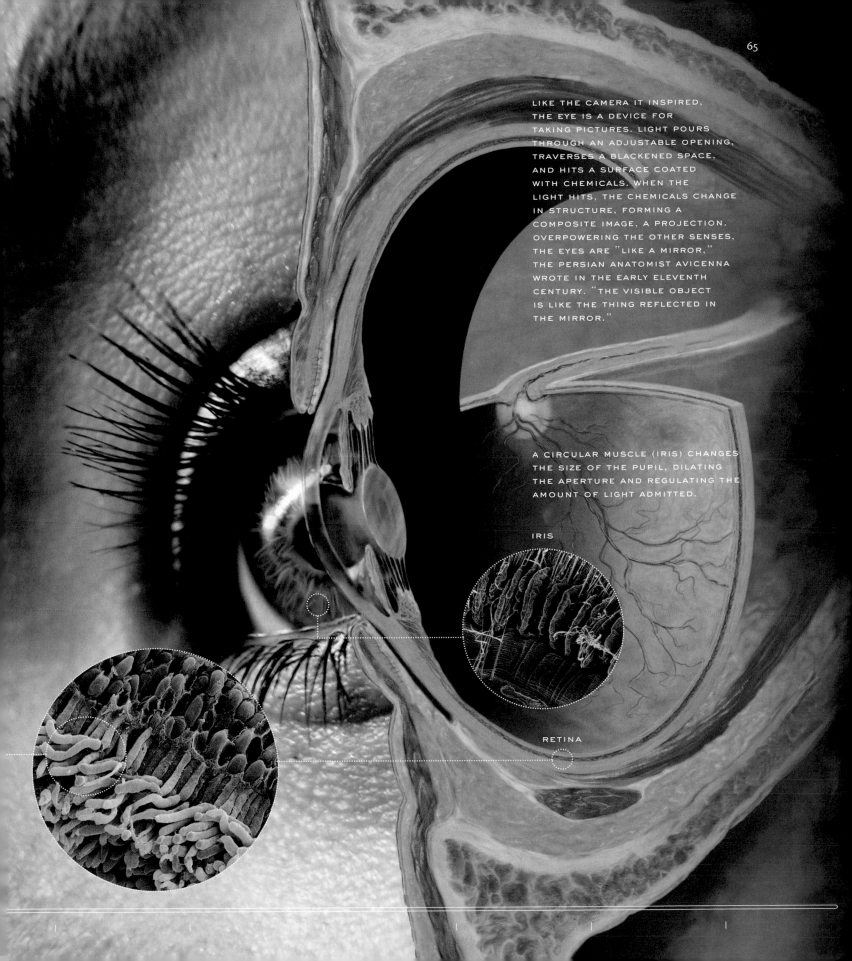

LIKE THE CAMERA IT INSPIRED, THE EYE IS A DEVICE FOR TAKING PICTURES. LIGHT POURS THROUGH AN ADJUSTABLE OPENING, TRAVERSES A BLACKENED SPACE, AND HITS A SURFACE COATED WITH CHEMICALS. WHEN THE LIGHT HITS, THE CHEMICALS CHANGE IN STRUCTURE, FORMING A COMPOSITE IMAGE, A PROJECTION. OVERPOWERING THE OTHER SENSES, THE EYES ARE "LIKE A MIRROR," THE PERSIAN ANATOMIST AVICENNA WROTE IN THE EARLY ELEVENTH CENTURY. "THE VISIBLE OBJECT IS LIKE THE THING REFLECTED IN THE MIRROR."

A CIRCULAR MUSCLE (IRIS) CHANGES THE SIZE OF THE PUPIL, DILATING THE APERTURE AND REGULATING THE AMOUNT OF LIGHT ADMITTED.

IRIS

RETINA

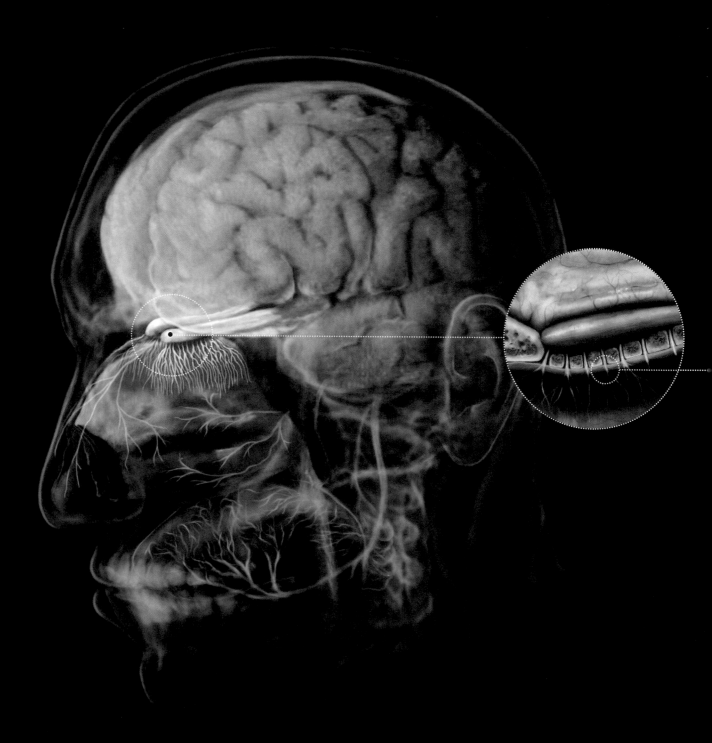

THE NOSE KNOWS

With each breath we take, a chemical air-filtration system located above and behind the nostrils identifies odor molecules and tells us how we ought to feel about them. As air enters the nasal cavity, millions of tall, slim cells, jammed together in a thumbnail-sized patch near the roof, sort out more than 10,000 different odors, at concentrations as low as one part in 30 billion. Many of these olfactory sensory cells have 10 to 20 tentaclelike hairs sticking downward into the watery mucus that coats the inner lining of the cavity. Swirling like sea anemones in a tide, the hairs (cilia) sweep up molecules dissolving in the mucus.

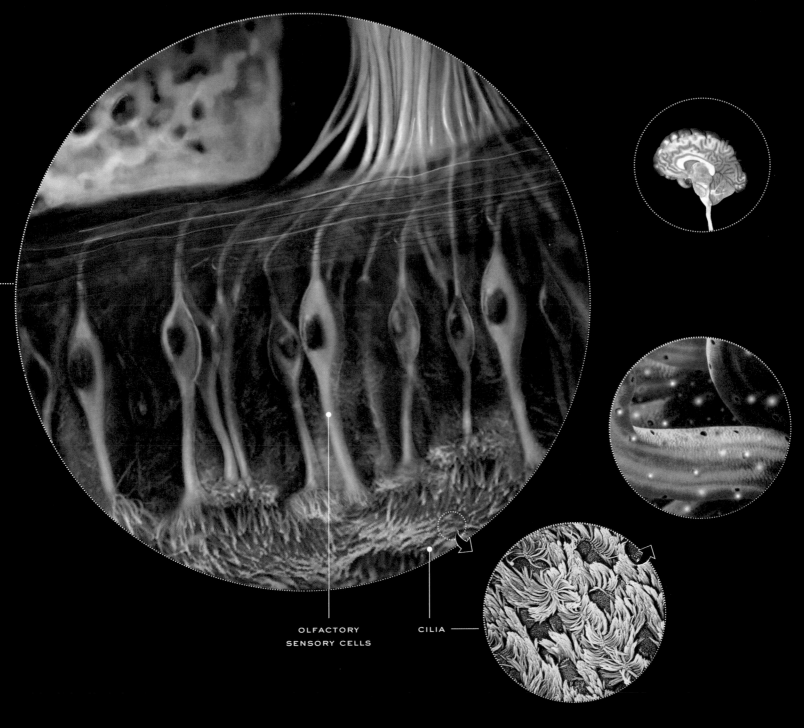

OLFACTORY
SENSORY CELLS

CILIA ——

Nerve signals triggered by these exchanges are bundled together and partly sorted in the olfactory bulbs which protrude like Q-Tips from the midbrain, where memories are "tagged" with feelings. The most direct of the senses, smell draws its power to evoke deep-seated emotions from linking so directly to the limbic system, the primitive junction where, in higher animals, lust, fear, memory, and aromatic arousal converge.

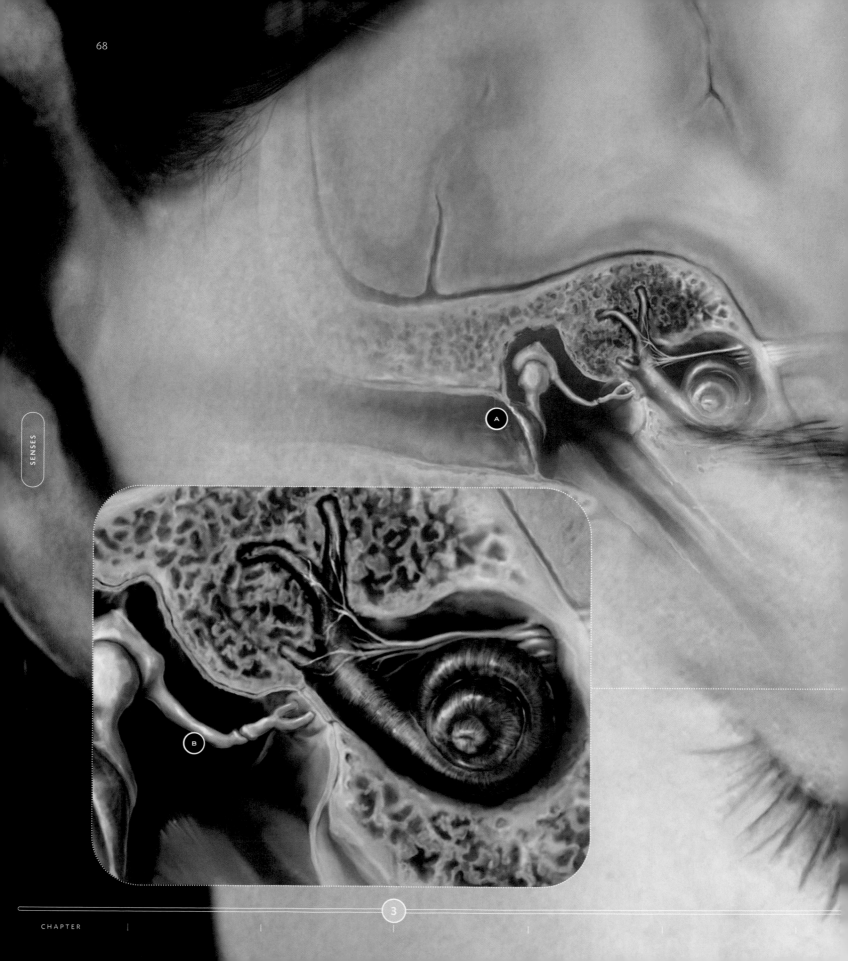

The auditory pathway, Ackerman writes, "looks something like a maniacal miniature golf course, with curlicues, branches, roundabouts, relays, levers, hydraulics and feedback loops"; or else "a contraption some ingenious plumber has put together from spare parts." Either way, Rube Goldberg could only marvel in disgust. Rather than using maximum effort to achieve minimal results, as Goldberg's cartoon inventions did, the ear translates sound waves into fluid waves, then electrical impulses, with astonishing efficiency: 99.9 percent of the sound energy transmitted into the tiny snail-like cochlea, which contains the organ of hearing, is conserved. The energy doesn't have to enter through the ear. Thomas Edison, who invented the first phonograph despite being nearly deaf, vetted pianists for early recording sessions by biting on the leg of the piano and listening to them through his teeth.

SOUND MACHINE

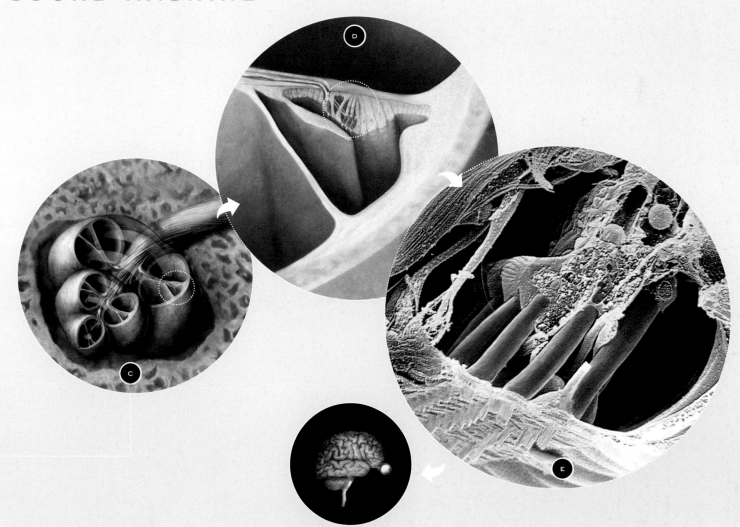

With so much moving in the world, torrents of vibrations rush at us from all around. The outer ear funnels them into a short tube ending at a fanlike drumhead (the eardrum) (A), which vibrates with them, which in turn relays the vibrations across a trio of hinged bones (B), the last of which (the smallest bone in the body) looks like a stirrup and taps like a piston-operated telegraph key on a window into the inner ear.

There the waves cross from air to liquid. The cochlea (c) is subdivided into 3 fluid-filled chambers, spiraling in parallel around a bony core. A spiral within a spiral, the organ of Corti (the hearing organ) (D) contains thousands of bristle-coated hair cells arranged in rows (E). When the fluid vibrates, the hairs move, exciting nerve cells, which send impulses to the brain, which interprets them as sounds.

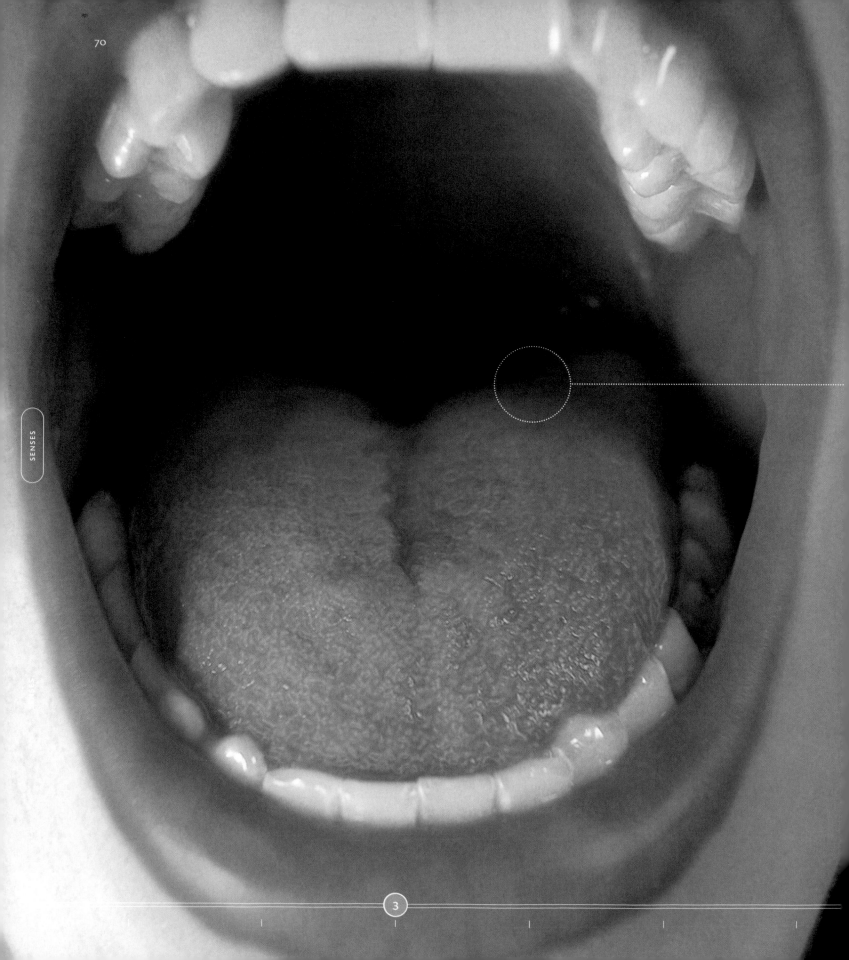

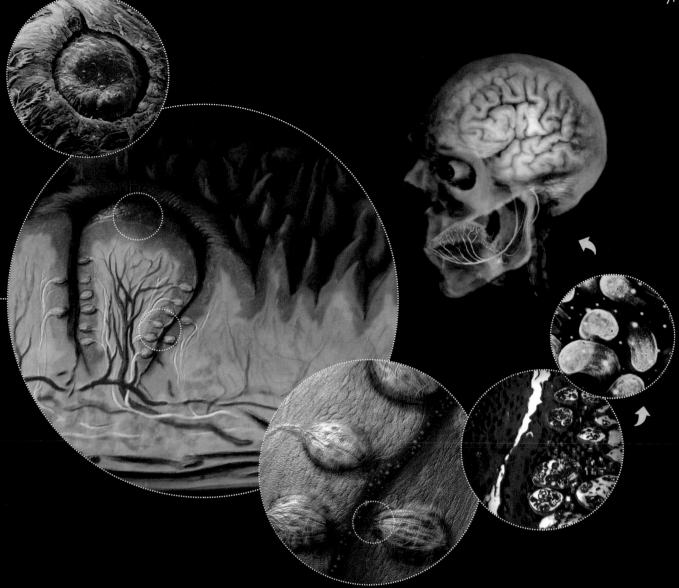

M M M M M M M , O O O O O O O O O O , Y C C H H H H H H

The Rolling Stones' Sticky Fingers logo, an exaggeratedly receptive tongue and mouth, tells the story.

Chemicals in food, liquids, or anything else passing the lips are quickly dissolved in liquid so they can be scanned by taste sensors on the tongue, palate, epiglottis, and throat, which classify them as either sweet, sour, salty, or bitter. Organized horizontally from the tip back—sweet first, because we need the energy stored in sugar molecules to live—legions of taste buds carpet the tongue. Onion shaped, each bud (cutaway

cycle) contains pods of elongated cells on which tiny hairs at the tip mingle with saliva that enters through a pore. As chemicals wash in, receptor molecules in the cells identify them, sending the information to the brain via 2 pairs of cranial nerves. The more you stick your tongue out, the more receptors you expose. Salacious, yes. Offensive, probably. But also an effective cartoon of the taste regions.

More subtle tastes occur when flavors blend and are aided by smells and other associated stimuli.

MIRRORED IN NATURE

The writer Paul Valéry, wondering about the enormous variety of seashells—their helices, spirals, bulbs, and concavities—compared the "making" of human beings with the slow, continuous formation that is the "making" of nature. Biological manufacturing patterns—blueprints—are widely copied: grooved cellular channels in the eye that resemble mushroom gills; the spiral of the ear's hearing chamber shares its shape with a snail shell; the tongue's spiny taste buds look remarkably like caterpillar spines. Up close everything looks like something else.

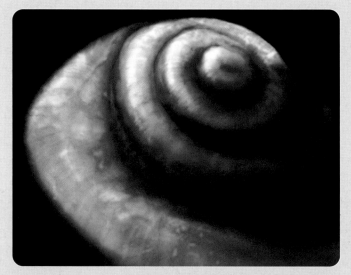

COCHLEA: INNER EAR HEARING MECHANISM

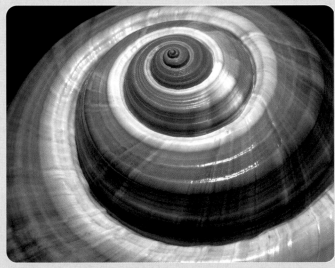

SNAIL SHELL

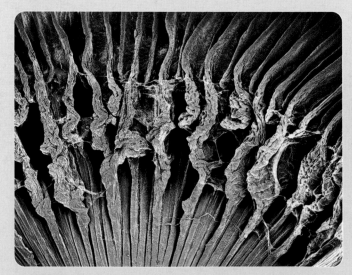

CILIARY BODY OF EYE

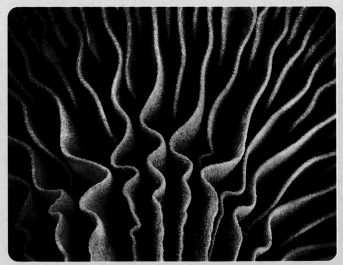

MUSHROOM GILLS

Though natural patterns reappear throughout sensory structures, occasionally too much is made of what these markings may tell us. The iris, a sphincter, is believed by followers of the "science" of iridology to reveal a "map of the whole body." Like foot reflexology charts, iridology charts divide the body into zones, and practitioners study site-specific changes in color, shape, and texture—orange in the digestive zone indicating a predisposition to diabetes, for instance; or a black speck indicating that your appendix has been surgically removed.

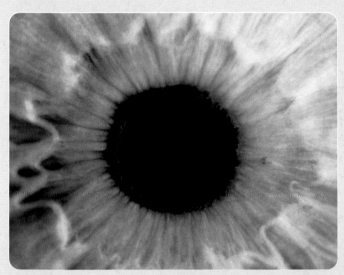

IRIS

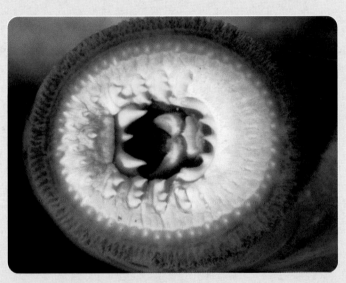

MOUTH PARTS OF A PACIFIC LAMPREY

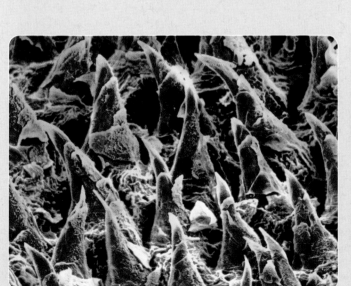

TONGUE SURFACE

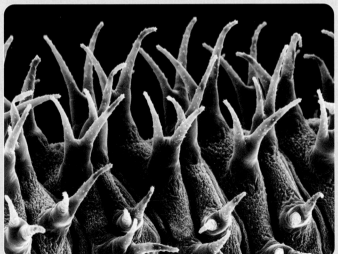

CATERPILLAR SPINES

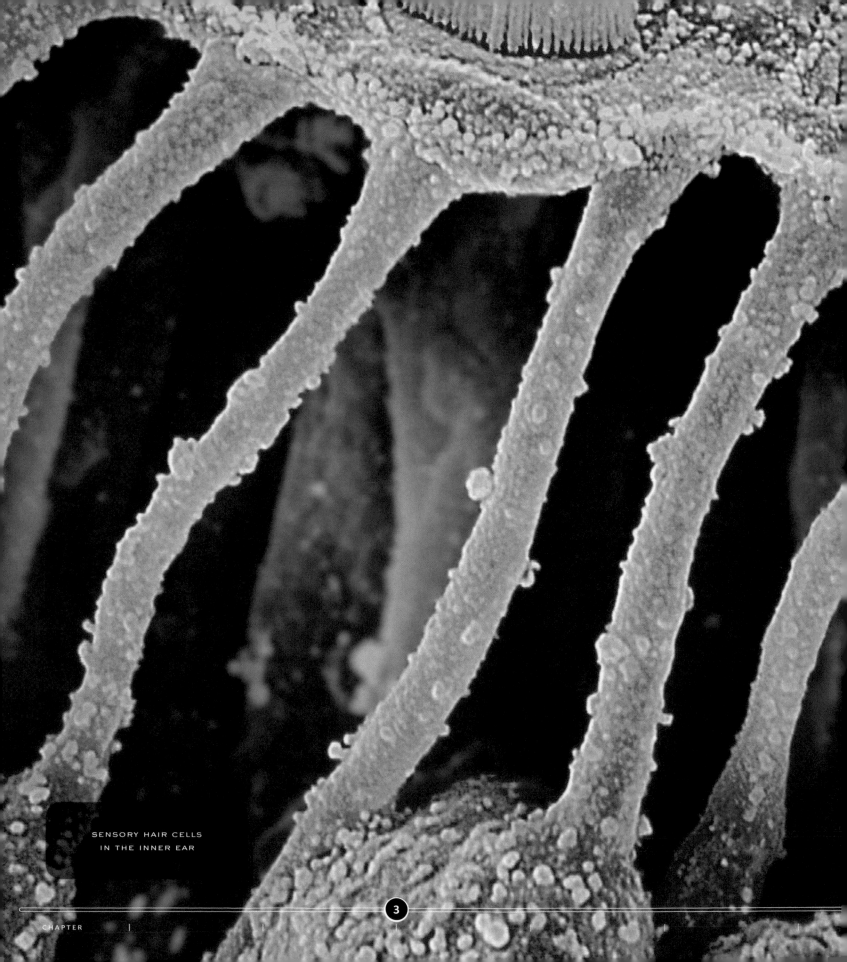

SENSORY HAIR CELLS
IN THE INNER EAR

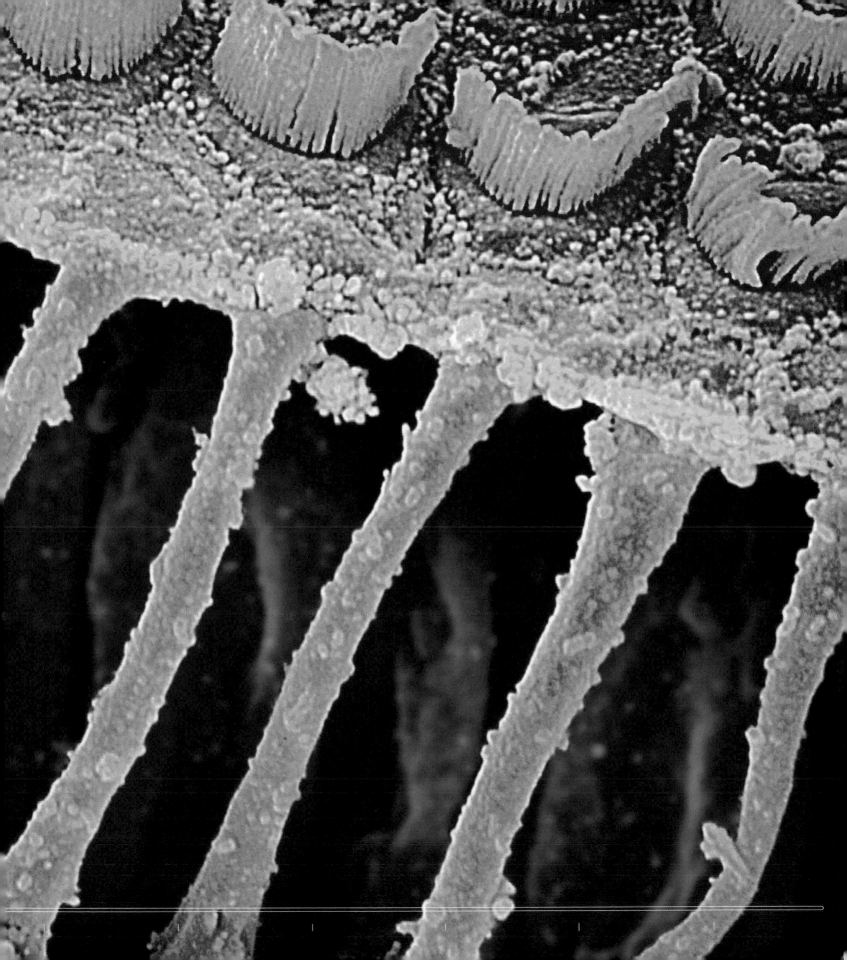

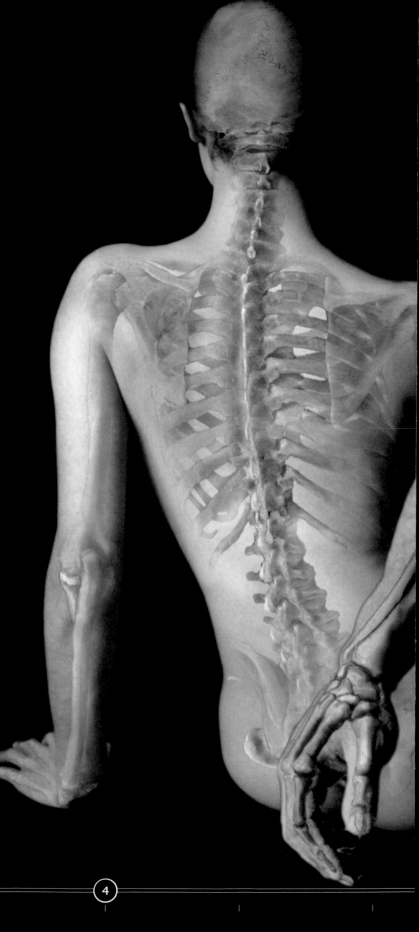

. . . your bones,
round rulers, round nudgers, round poles,
numb nubkins, the sword of sugar.
I feel the skull, Mr. Skeleton, living its
own life in its own skin.
—Anne Sexton

structural
framework

(skeletal system)

Twice as tough as granite for withstanding compression forces, 4 times more resilient than concrete in standing up to stretching, about 5 times as light as steel. As D'Arcy Thompson observed, bone is an architect's dream, a building material so malleable that it can be hammered into any shape, so versatile that when it's assembled into a light and durable framework it can execute and withstand complex mechanical movements, and so strong that it gives shape to and stiffens the whole human form without buckling. Not simply exquisite, as all great architecture must be, the edifice of the human skeleton is a perfect diagram of the lines of stress, tension, and compression involved in bearing the loaded structure—*us*—through a century or more of activity.

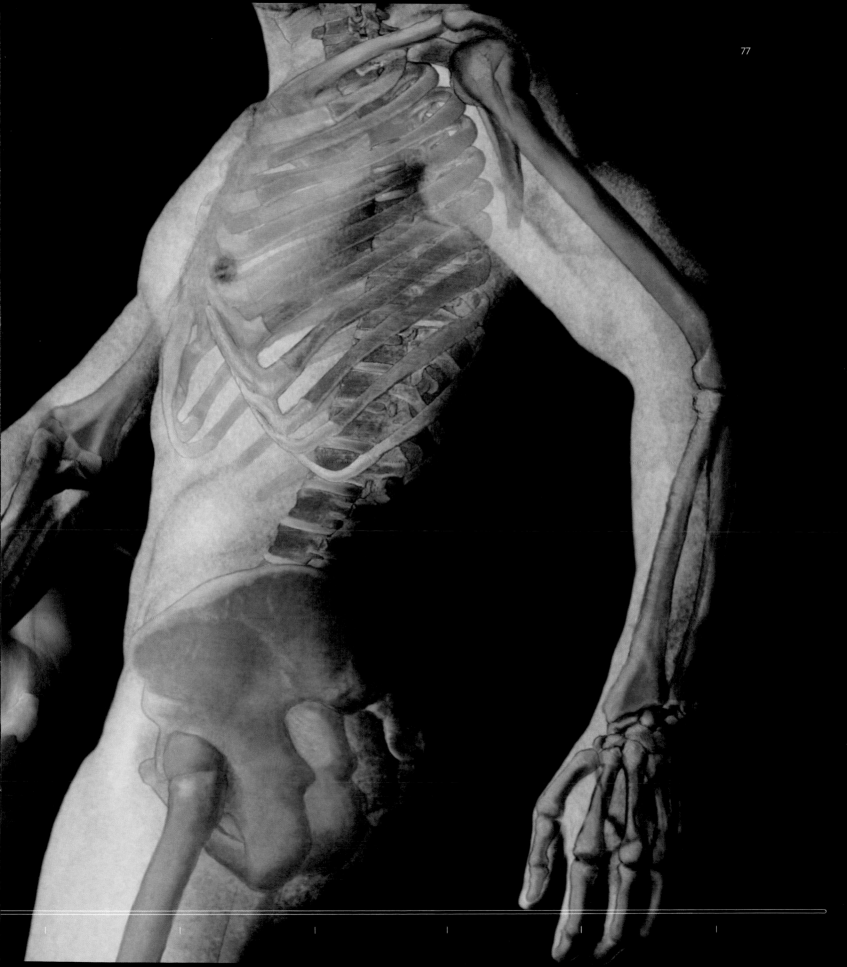

In the first stage of erecting a building or bridge, an initial frame is assembled of hot-rolled, carbon steel rods (rebars). Cement is then poured around them, forming a tight union to create a structure that can withstand rocking motions while maintaining strength. Without the steel rods, the cement would be too brittle, and would fracture easily; without the cement, the rebars would be too weak to support the overall load, and would bend.

So it is with bone. At 6 weeks after conception, rods of collagen, tightly wound chains of long protein molecules, become the body's incipient rebars, laying down a model for the full skeleton. Within 2 months, minerals from the blood crystallize and surround the rods, hardening like cement, although the bones still aren't connected at the joints. At

birth, the bones have ossified enough to support the body, but it will take another year or more before complex joint mechanisms tie them all together to deliver enough strength and flexibility to permit, say, toddling.

The structural matrix of bone—a tight, interactive mix of protein and minerals—makes it a better building material than alloys and composites, but the true brilliance of its design is that it *lives*. The skeleton, like any living system, breaks down and renews itself continually. As the body grows to adulthood, it adapts its shape and proportions to match the demands of maturation. When bones break, they mend themselves. Growing outward from the middle of the shaft, the long bones that give the body its adult contours continue to grow until the age of 17 to 21.

ERECTOR SET

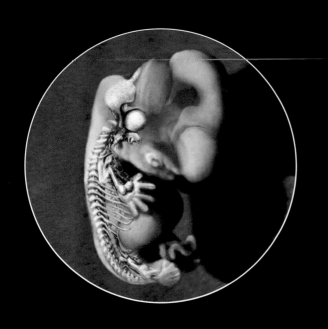

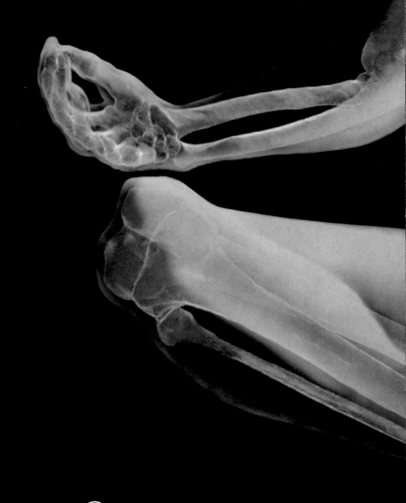

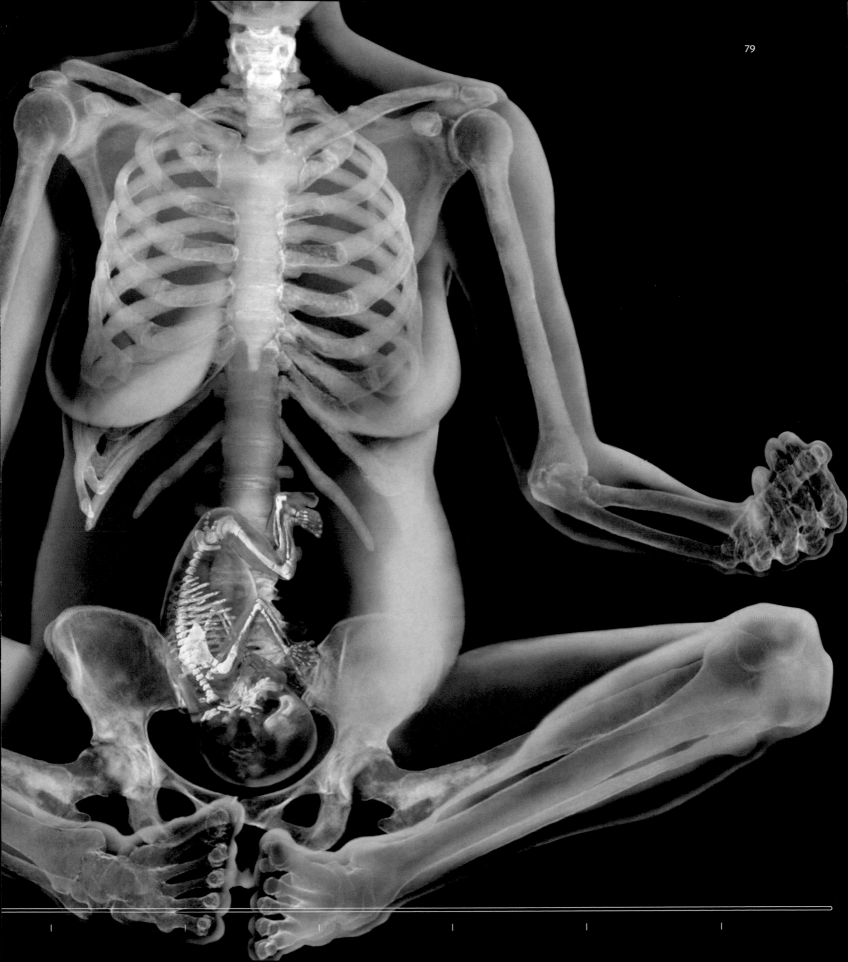

Brilliantly engineered to distribute force, the living skeleton not only bears the body's load and enables movement but also stores minerals, protects internal organs, and, in its spongy interiors, houses the main bloodworks. Grayish in color, this flexible armature pivots along a central axis (the spine), which bends and turns and is attached to rings of bones (girdles) that connect it to the limbs. Arms and legs share the same fundamental structure—1 long bone, 2 shorter ones, and a clawlike assembly of yet smaller ones, all hinged by freely moveable joints.

SUPPORT AND MOVEMENT

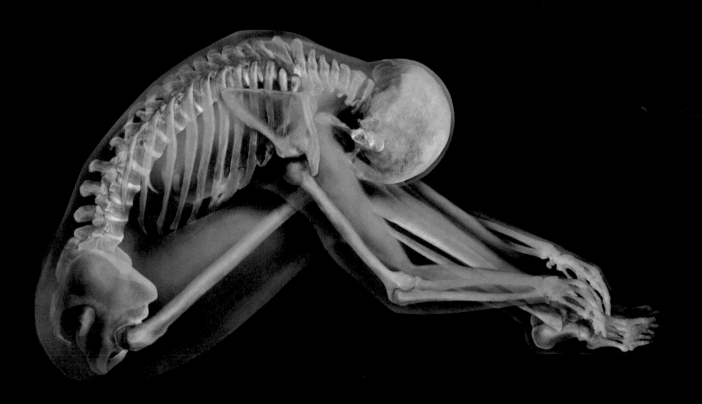

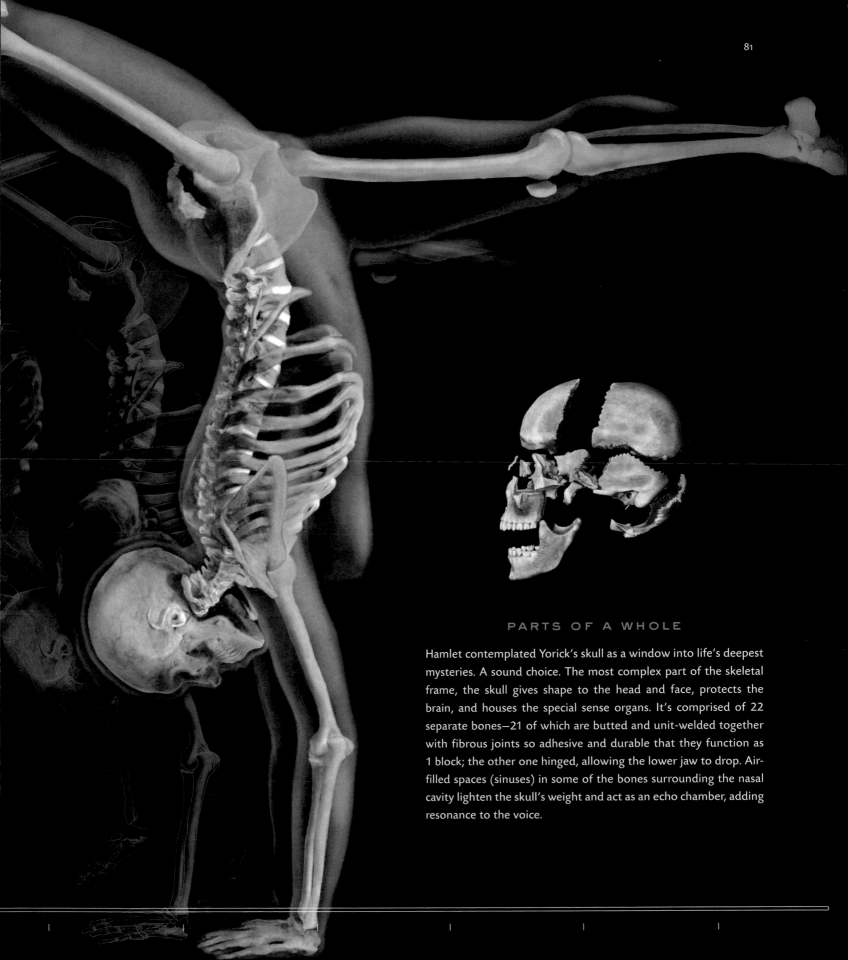

PARTS OF A WHOLE

Hamlet contemplated Yorick's skull as a window into life's deepest mysteries. A sound choice. The most complex part of the skeletal frame, the skull gives shape to the head and face, protects the brain, and houses the special sense organs. It's comprised of 22 separate bones—21 of which are butted and unit-welded together with fibrous joints so adhesive and durable that they function as 1 block; the other one hinged, allowing the lower jaw to drop. Air-filled spaces (sinuses) in some of the bones surrounding the nasal cavity lighten the skull's weight and act as an echo chamber, adding resonance to the voice.

A bone's shape dictates what it does and vice versa. Long bones raise and lower as levers, short bones bridge spaces, flat bones shield and protect, irregular bones like the vertebrae and ilium (1 of the bones in each half of the pelvis) serve as customized flanks, flanges, collars, and crowns.

Sesame seed–shaped bones embedded in soft tissue (like the patella) cap vulnerable areas. The structural matrix of each bone—how cells align throughout the tissue—is arranged to transmit compression and tension forces optimally within its particular shape.

FORM FOLLOWS FUNCTION

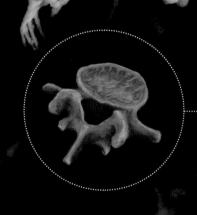

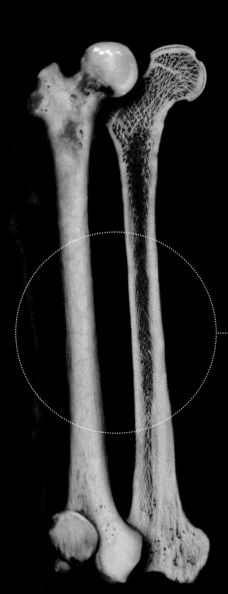

LONG BONE (FEMUR)

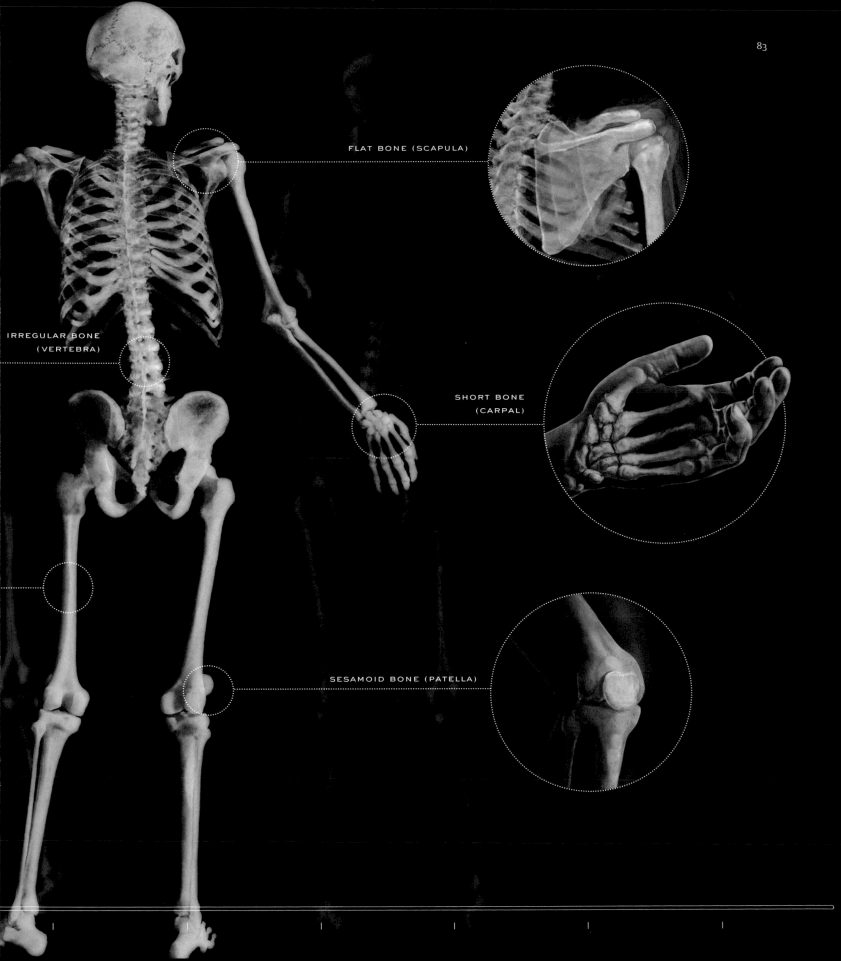

FLAT BONE (SCAPULA)

IRREGULAR BONE
(VERTEBRA)

SHORT BONE
(CARPAL)

SESAMOID BONE (PATELLA)

STRUCTURAL CORE

The combination of strength, flexibility, and armor-cladding is achieved by an S-shaped stack of variously shaped irregular bones, interspersed with springy disks of tough cartilage. The disks act like ball bearings, absorbing forces of up to several hundred pounds per square inch during strenuous exercise. To keep the column from overtwisting like Popeye's girl, Olive Oyl, or bending so much that our heads snap backwards or pitch into our laps, the vertebrae are equipped with "processes"—outgrowths—that link to form hinges and "facet joints," rounded ends fitted to matching hollows that work like "hinge-pin" doorstops, limiting movement within a prescribed arc. The S shape adds resilience and maintains a balanced center of gravity.

Much of a man's character will be found betokened in his backbone . . .
A thin joist of a spine never yet upheld a full and noble soul.
—Herman Melville

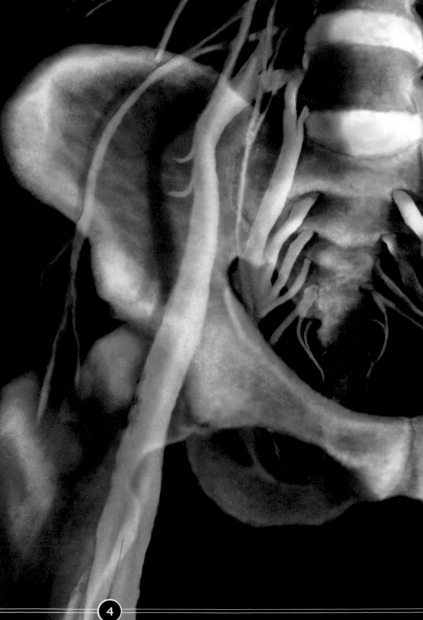

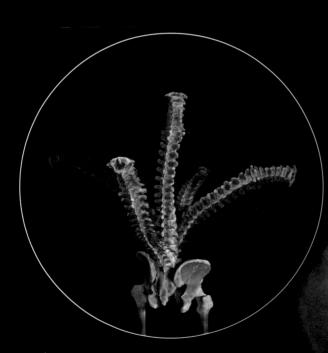

MORE THAN THE SUM OF ITS PARTS, THE SPINAL COLUMN HOLDS OUR HEADS AND UPPER BODIES UPRIGHT, LIKE A CENTRAL PILLAR, WHILE ALSO ALLOWING THE BODY TO BEND AND TWIST. MEANWHILE, IT PROTECTS THE SPINAL CORD.

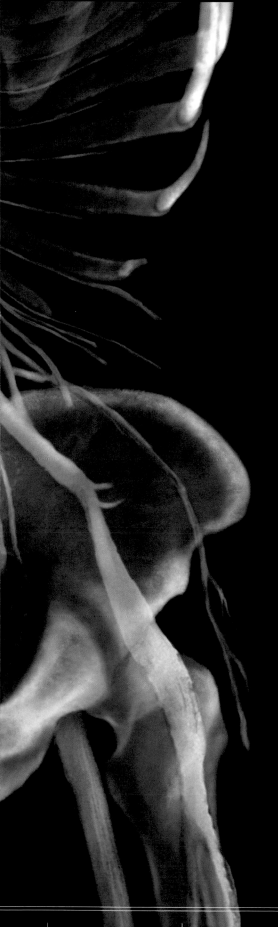

DIFFERENT REGIONS, DIFFERENT SHAPES

Each section of the spine is designed for a specific purpose. The flattened vertebrae on top support the head and neck; those behind the chest anchor the rib cage; and those at the base are thick, wide, and strong, to bear weight and provide stability.

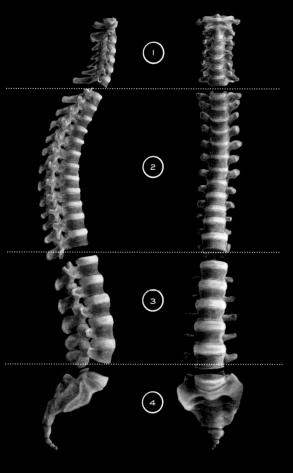

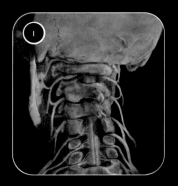

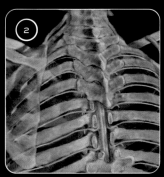

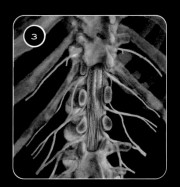

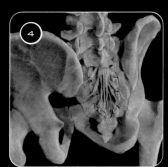

GENDER DIFFERENCES

The size of the female skull is, on average, $^4/_5$ that of the male, and a woman's facial skeleton is generally less angular than a man's; less square in the chin, less severe in the jaw (A), more convex in the forehead. In "gender-confirming facial surgery"—the remodeling of the face's bony architecture in people who've had sex changes—particular attention is paid to the area of the orbits, the pyramid–shaped cavities that house and protect the eyeballs (B). These appear higher, more rounded, and relatively large in the female skull, providing what one study on gender and expression calls "the soft and 'sincere' look of the feminine face."

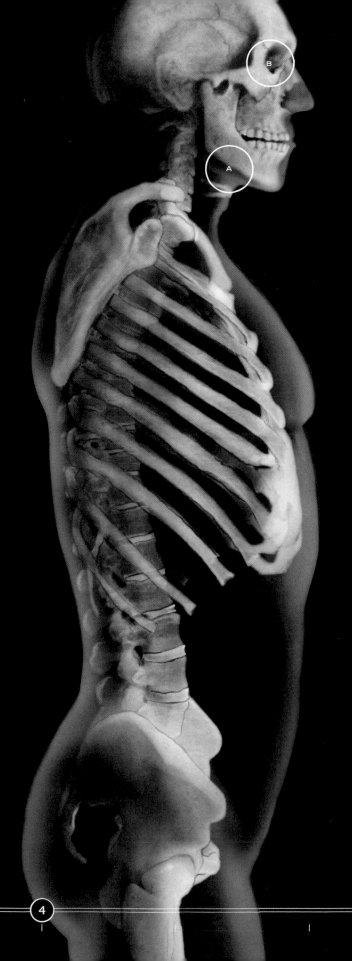

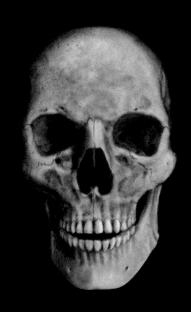

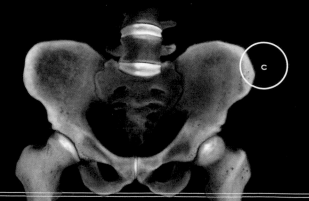

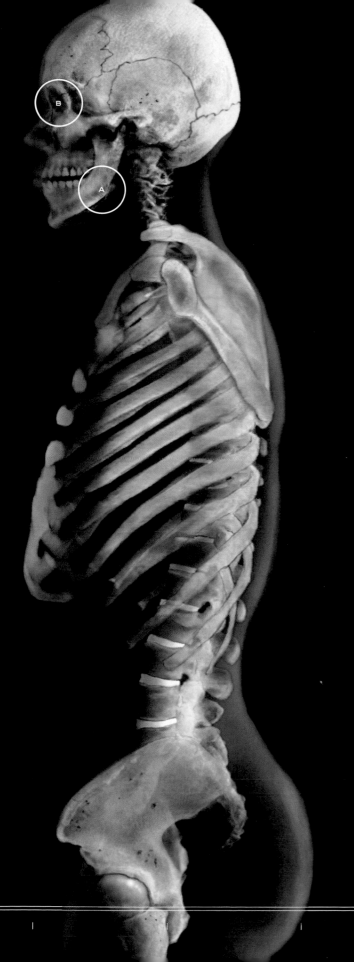

Women have narrower shoulders and their arms are usually shorter, meaning they have less leverage in throwing. Similarly, their hips are wider (c) (the result of a more open pelvis, for childbearing), which increases the angle between the pelvis and thighbone and makes it harder for them to raise their knees as high as men, or push on the ground with as much force, while running. On the other hand, lower hips and narrower shoulders create a lower center of gravity, making women's bodies more stable.

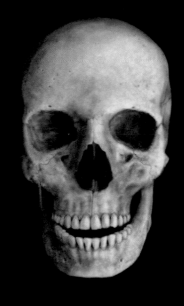

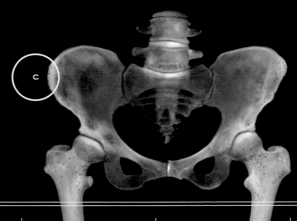

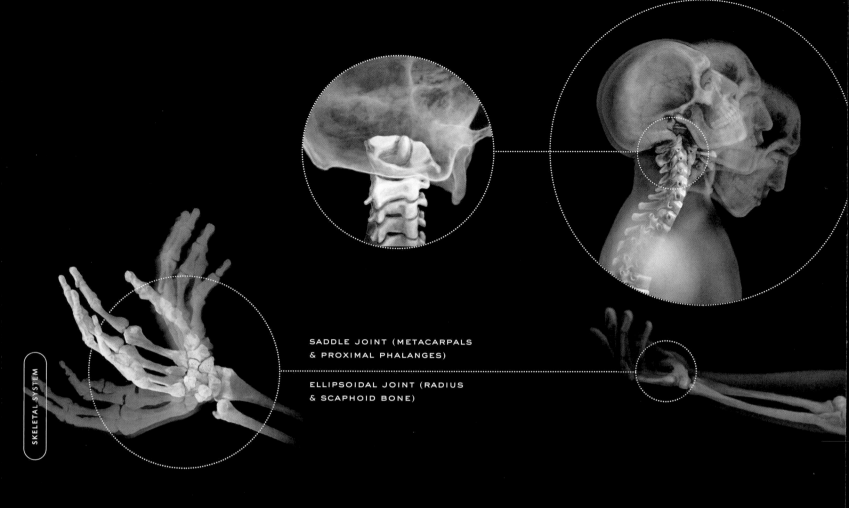

SADDLE JOINT (METACARPALS
& PROXIMAL PHALANGES)

ELLIPSOIDAL JOINT (RADIUS
& SCAPHOID BONE)

RANGE OF MOTION

Exemplifying the idea of body-as-machine are the synovial joints—the long-lasting, lubricated bearings between bones that allow them to slide by each other in passing. Bones like those in the shoulder, where a spherical head fits into a bowl-shaped cavity, allow movement in 2 planes plus some twisting (which, in combination, allow us to scratch our own backs). Ellipsoidal (saddle) joints, like those at the base of the thumb, fit 2 spoon-shaped bone ends snugly together to form a pivot (making it possible, at the piano, to scoot the thumbs under the hands).

With both concave and convex areas, the bones can rock back and forth and side to side, but have limited rotation.

Like, say, car transmissions and door hinges, synovial joints are designed to ease the transfer of mechanical forces while cutting down on friction and resisting wear. Encapsulated in its own flexible bag, each such joint contains a waterproof cavity in which smooth bone ends are cushioned by a shock absorber of pearl-smooth elastic material and "oiled" by the thick, slippery fluid (synovia) for which it's named.

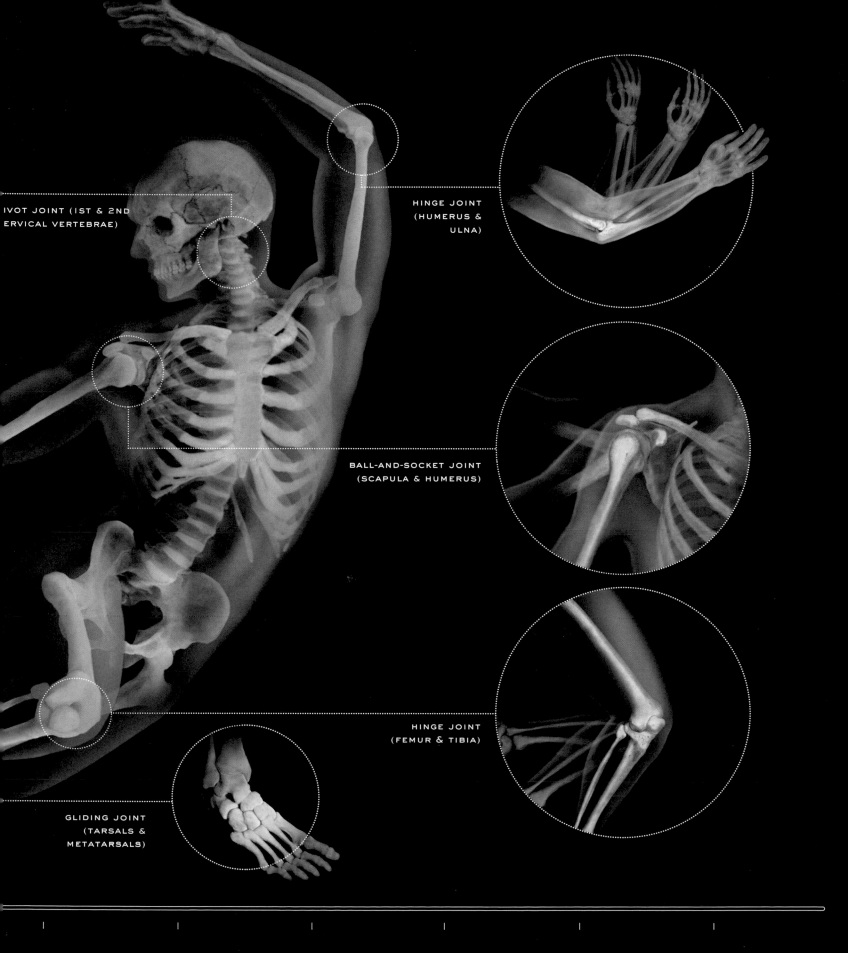

IVOT JOINT (1ST & 2ND
ERVICAL VERTEBRAE)

HINGE JOINT
(HUMERUS &
ULNA)

BALL-AND-SOCKET JOINT
(SCAPULA & HUMERUS)

HINGE JOINT
(FEMUR & TIBIA)

GLIDING JOINT
(TARSALS &
METATARSALS)

CONNECTORS AND CUSHIONS

As a construction material, strandlike collagen is extraordinarily versatile. Mixed with minerals, collagen rods harden into bone, much as bricks and mortar interact to form a wall. Without minerals, the fibers assemble into different patterns and matrices to create the strong, elastic structures—connective tissue—that tie bones and other structural units together into working mechanisms.

Firm, compact cartilage makes up the framework of discrete structures such as the nose, ears, and trachea; sculpts and sleekens the ends of bones; cushions joints; and forms sheaths and capsules like those surrounding the knee. When collagen is bundled and packed together like twisted rope, it becomes sinew—living cables—strapping bone to muscle and muscle to muscle. Packed in layers or sheets and interwoven with elastin, a protein that can stretch and contract, it becomes resilient like a bungee cord, or like the ligaments that join bone to bone.

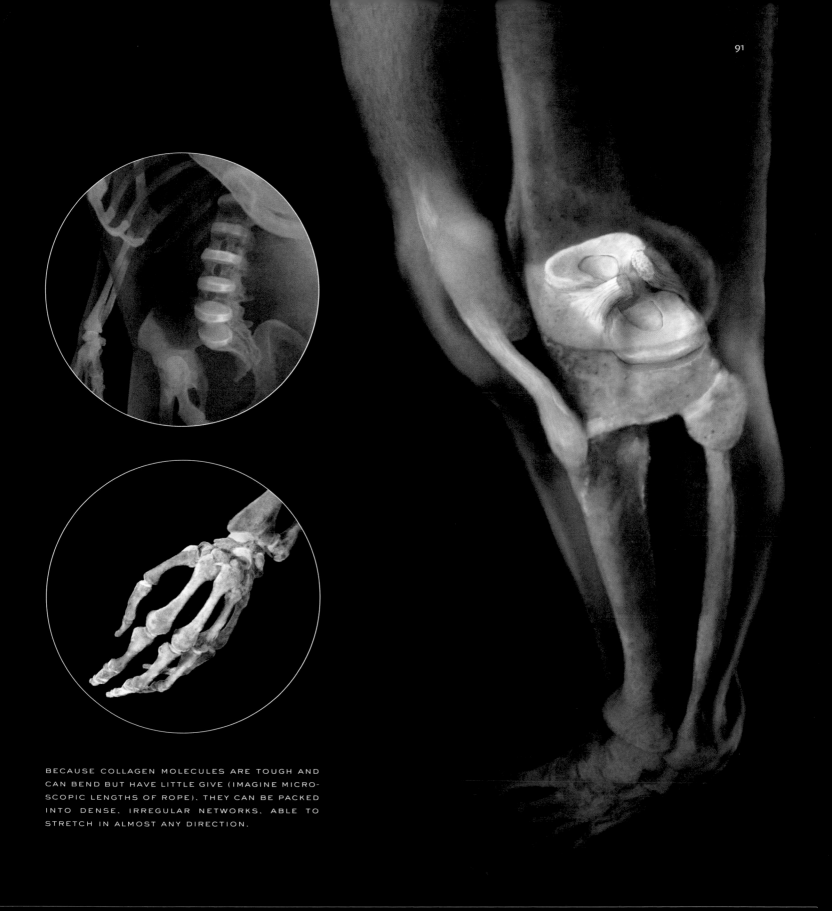

BECAUSE COLLAGEN MOLECULES ARE TOUGH AND
CAN BEND BUT HAVE LITTLE GIVE (IMAGINE MICRO-
SCOPIC LENGTHS OF ROPE), THEY CAN BE PACKED
INTO DENSE, IRREGULAR NETWORKS, ABLE TO
STRETCH IN ALMOST ANY DIRECTION.

As late as 1620, a learned Scottish physician could lecture his students, "Bone is . . . generated out of semen, fat and earth by the power of heat and the innate spirit."

It wasn't until 70 years later, when the English physiologist Clopton Havers first described the microscopic structure of bones, that their principle organizing features were identified.

The underlying structure of bone consists of living cells and protein fibers wrapped around layers of hard mineral salts. Long bones like the femur consist of concentric rings of these mixtures, ranging in texture from corallike to compact or wood-like, to rock-hard—a pattern of cylinders packed within cylinders laced with wormholes. Surrounding the fat storehouse of the inner marrow, the spongy, innermost cylinder (A) is a matrix of rigid struts, which take some of the load that the bone has to bear while leaving space for production of red blood cells.

Havers discovered that the middle, compact layer is made up of concentric bony tubes (B) bundled like logs on a truck, each one laced with a system of canals containing blood vessels. Special holes, or pits, allow enough space for individual bone cells (C) to reside within, where they secrete bone salts needed for growth and repair. The cylinder's outer layer (D), called the cement line, attaches to the enamel-hard exterior shell, which is irrigated by blood vessels and innervated by neurons that can signal pain.

COMPOSITION

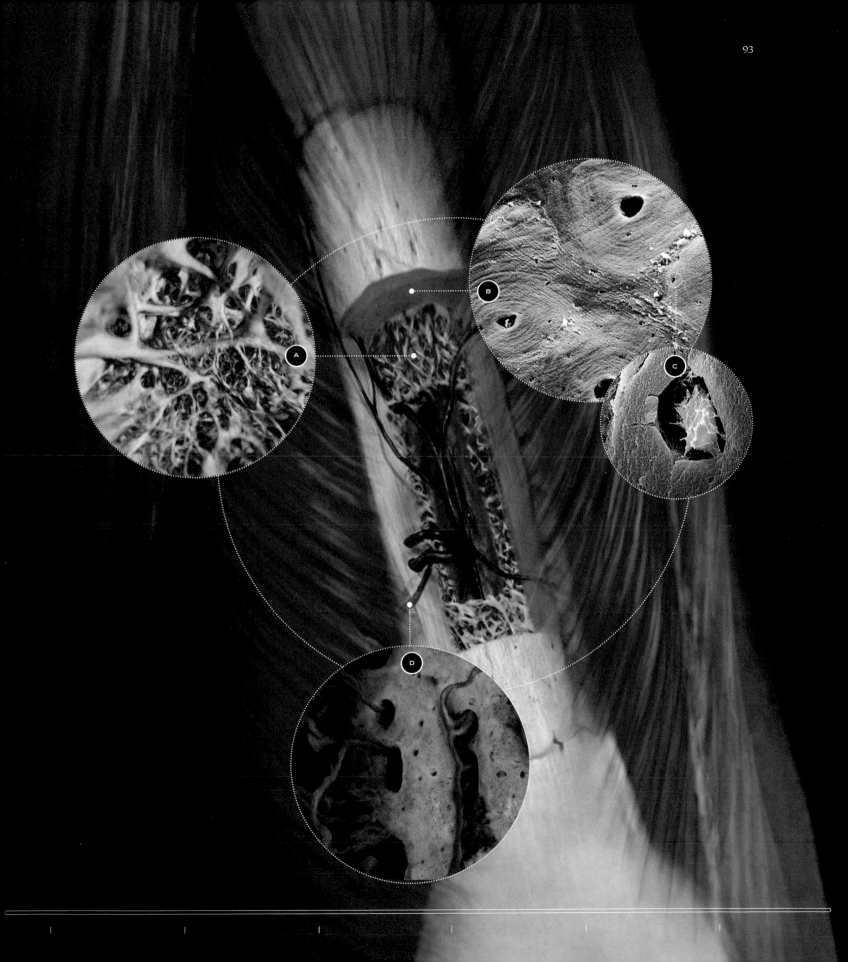

SKELETAL SYSTEM

MIRRORED IN NATURE

The spongy latticework of *cancellous* bone is typical of cubicle-like natural structures that house hives of activity, while the concentric, leeklike construction of cortical (hard) bone is built primarily to be strong, making it difficult for

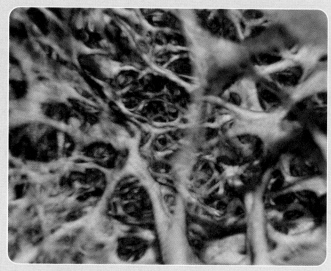

BONE MATRIX

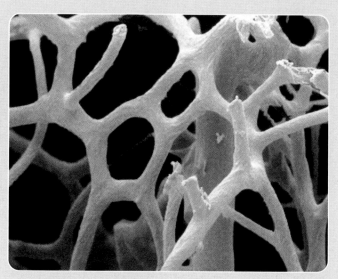

SALT WATER NATURAL SPONGE

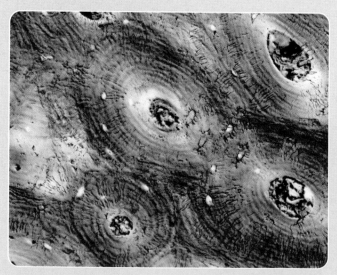

HARD BONE

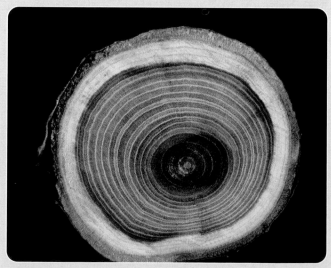

TREE GROWTH RINGS

cracks to spread. Collagen, which takes many forms, resembles the curly growth patterns of poplar wood and the fan-

ning array of small bones in the hand echo other skeletons in nature.

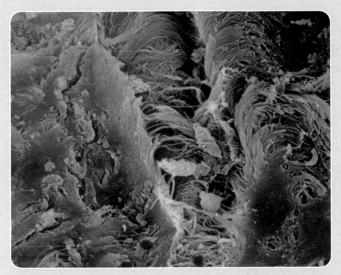

COLLAGEN IN BONE

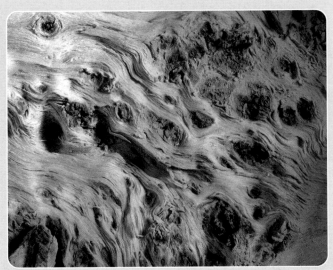

POPLAR WOOD

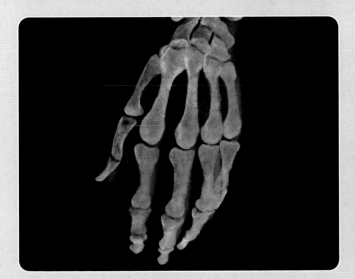

PHALANGES OF HAND

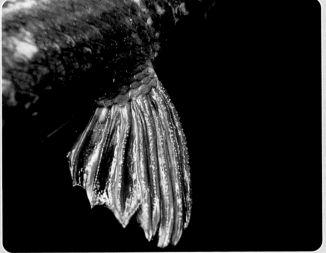

FISH FIN (COELACANTH)

COMPACT BONE IS COMPRISED OF SHEETS OF COMPACTED COLLAGEN FIBERS.

CHAPTER 4

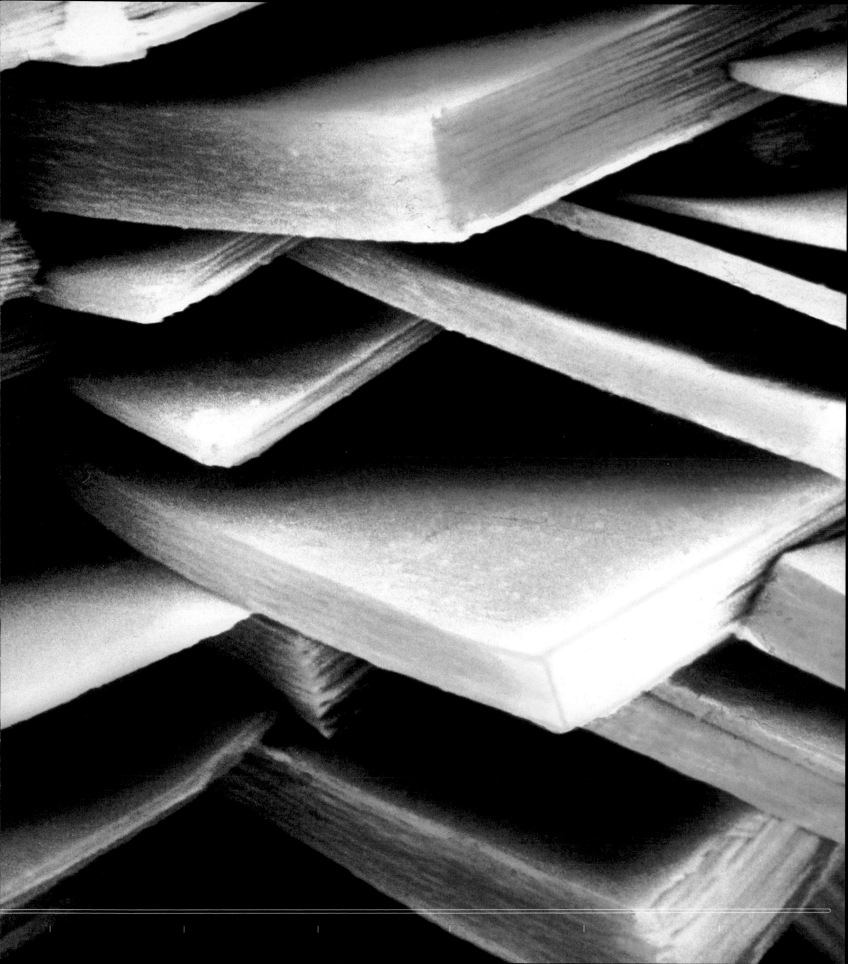

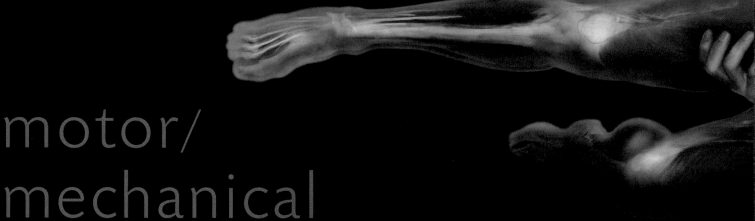

The power of locomotion is that which contracts and relaxes the muscles whereby the members and joints are moved, extended or flexed. This power reaches the limbs by way of the nerves and there are as many forms of power as there are of movement. Each muscle has its own peculiar purpose and it obeys the decree of the composite sense.
–Eleventh-century Persian anatomist Avicenna

motor/
mechanical

(muscular system)

The poetry of human motion lies under the skin, in the exquisite coordination of more than 600 individual pulling devices, a rigging of powerful elastic straps comprising about half the body's weight. Since the devices work one way only—by shortening, then returning to their original length—each muscle is partnered with an "antagonist" that pulls the same bone in the opposite direction. Teams of 30 or more muscles hoisting and stretching together can move, lift, and rotate bones in a group, engineering the body's major movements and postures.

Researchers have understood since the mid–nineteenth century that muscles are *chemicomechanical* devices: they convert chemical energy into work, like minuscule internal combustion engines. Muscle cells, their structural units, are long rods consisting of bundles of fibers that are themselves ganged "threads" of hair-thin microfibers. In the early 1930s a German chemist, Karl Lohmann, identified the universal fuel that powers them—ATP, adenosine triphosphate, an energy-rich compound. When ATP breaks down in the cell and releases its fuel, these microfibers attach and slide past each other, as if pulling a rope line hand-over-hand. Repeated hundreds of times per second across thousands of filaments in each fiber, then over and over again across the whole fabric of stringy, resilient muscle tissue, this rapid cycling enables muscles to contract and relax.

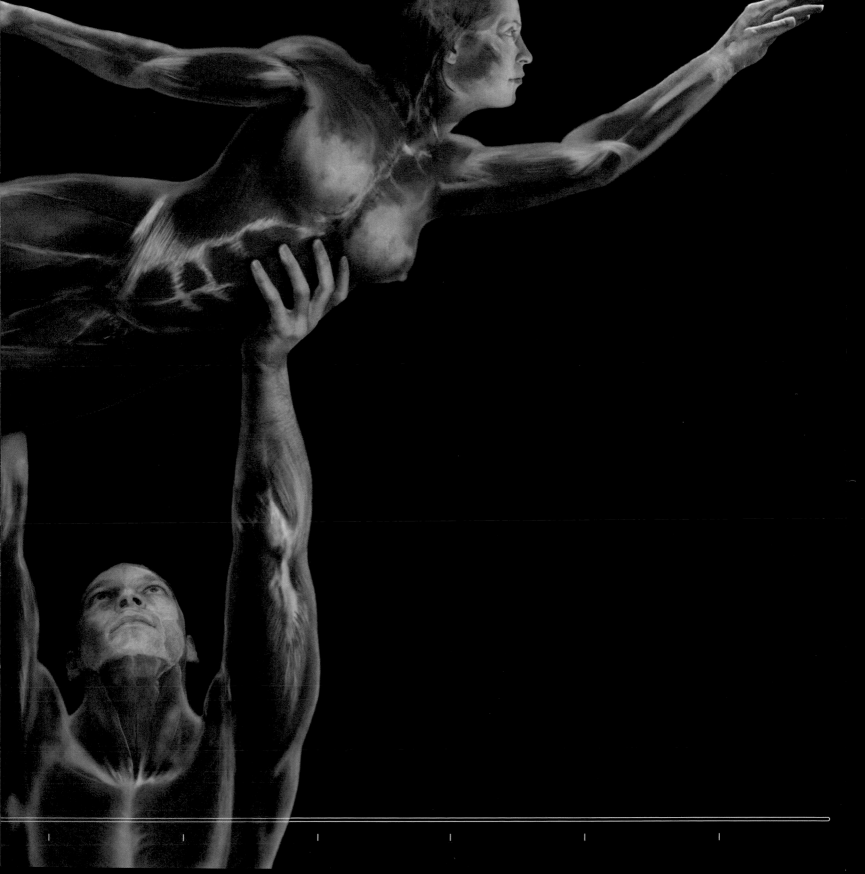

DEVELOPMENT

Three types of muscles start to organize by the end of the first month after conception—heart, gut, and voluntary. Four weeks later, all muscle blocks have appeared, as the heart partitions into chambers, the alimentary canal extends from the mouth to the intestines, and the limb buds emerge. By the middle of the second trimester, the heart recirculates about 25 quarts of blood through the body per day while the skeletal muscles develop strength, coordination, and reflex action—well before newborns will need them.

Although the system of skeletal (voluntary) muscles is fully laid down at birth, it takes several years for mature movement patterns to develop. Take gait, for instance—our manner of walking on 2 legs, which in adults involves shifting the body's weight smoothly over a narrow pivot point with minimal changes in the center of gravity and with what orthopedists call "reciprocal arm swing." All this must be learned—first by suppressing uncontrolled and chaotic primitive reflexes to bring the musculature firmly under the brain's control, then by many years of practice.

First, children toddle; their stance is wide, they walk on their heels, they're off balance, their hips rotate while their knees remain flexed, their arms are held in "high guard." By age 2, as the brain begins to integrate the movement of many joints and muscles, children's pelvises tilt less, 80 percent of them have begun to swing their arms, and the amount of time spent supported by a single leg increases to about one third. By age 3, most children have developed an adult pattern of joint angles, but it takes several more years of refinement and bone growth to achieve the same cadence, step length, and velocity as adults.

TYPE OF MUSCLE
(VOLUNTARY AND INVOLUNTARY)

Muscle tissue generally appears either "striped" or "unstriped" (smooth), reflecting, in the first case, the ability to be put into action and controlled by the will, and in the second, to be part of an automatic process like digestion. When we blink or swing a sledgehammer, ropelike cylindrical fibers, some up to a foot long, contract, helping to move parts of the body. When we swallow and breathe, sheets of tightly packed fibers rolled into tubes or sacs also contract, reducing the space inside them and moving a visceral process along.

The tissue of the heart, laced with a magnificent wiring system that takes nerve signals to the deepest regions and jolts them into rhythmic pulsing, is a special case. Smaller than those of other striped muscles, cardiac fibers contract and release automatically, about 100,000 times a day.

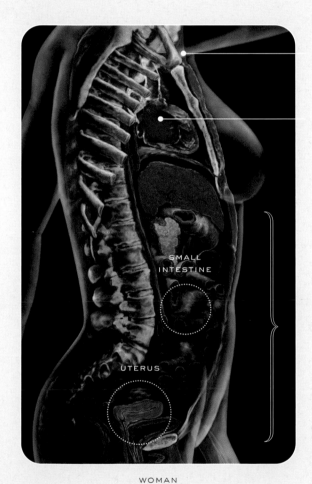

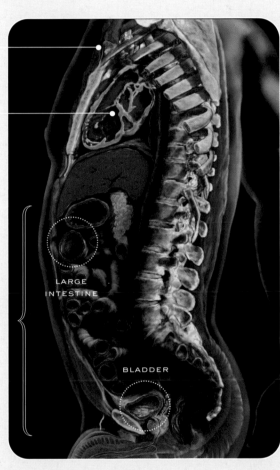

SKELETAL MUSCLE

CARDIAC MUSCLE

SMALL INTESTINE

LARGE INTESTINE

SMOOTH MUSCLE

UTERUS

BLADDER

WOMAN

MAN

GENDER DIFFERENCES

Men have fifty percent greater muscle mass, based on weight, than women, and muscle structures vary. Smaller-sized muscles are capable of exerting less force, which increases wear and breakage. Studies show, for instance, that women suffer up to 8 times more knee injuries in "pivot" sports, where knees may endure heavy turns, twists, and jerks. Less massive, their knee muscles often don't produce enough stiffness (without being specifically trained) to protect sensitive ligaments behind the kneecap.

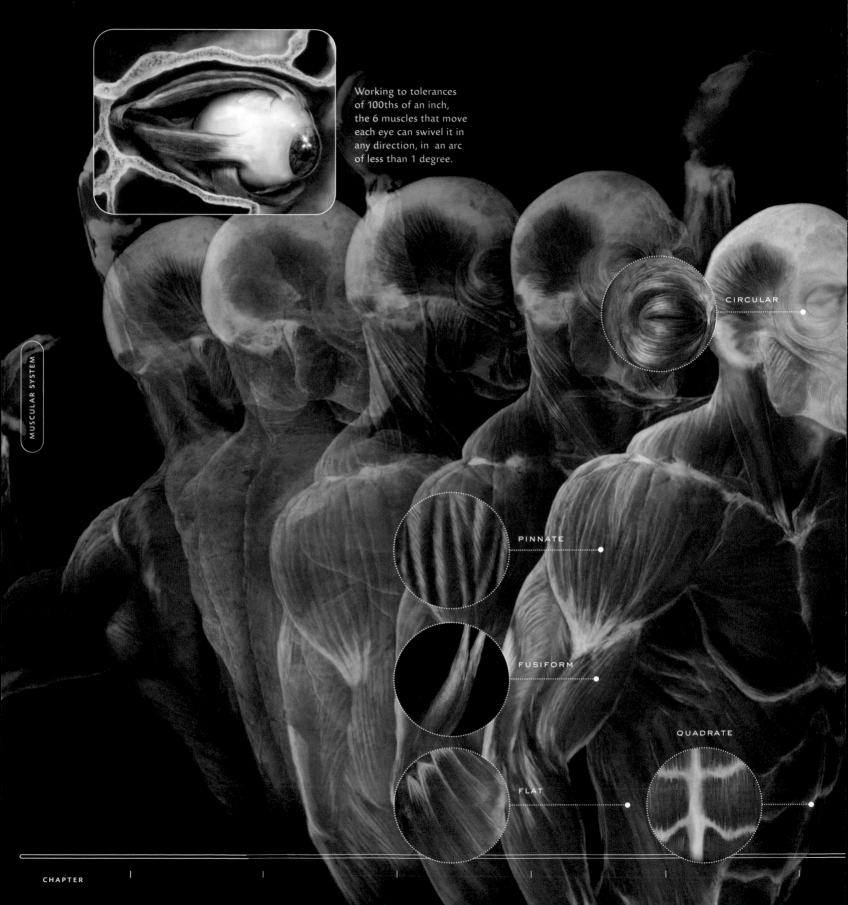

Working to tolerances
of 100ths of an inch,
the 6 muscles that move
each eye can swivel it in
any direction, in an arc
of less than 1 degree.

MUSCULAR SYSTEM

CIRCULAR

PINNATE

FUSIFORM

QUADRATE

FLAT

To boot a soccer ball, the leg works like a powerful 3-part lever. Muscle groups working with and against each other swing the thigh at the hip, pivot the lower leg at the knee, and tilt the foot at the ankle. The calf muscles pull on the heel bone to tilt the foot down while the opposing muscles in the shin pull on the front of the ankle and foot bones to raise the toes, thus multiplying the force and accuracy of the kick.

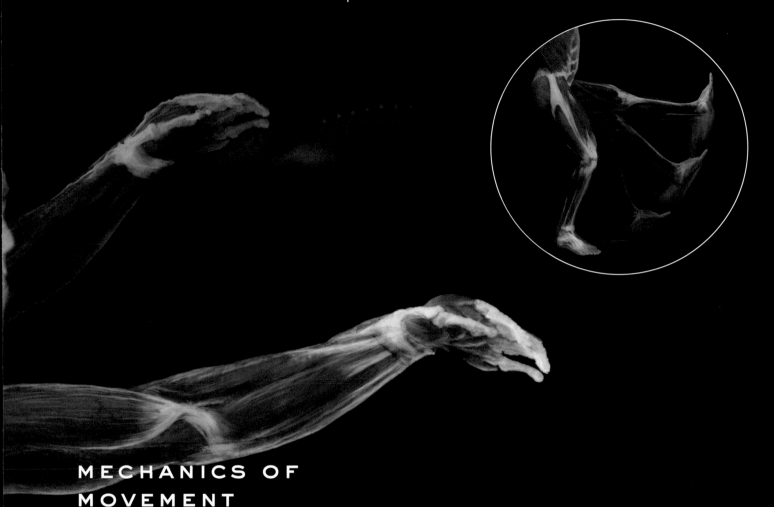

MECHANICS OF MOVEMENT

The task of throwing a football requires the body to become a catapult. Fancy footwork, a slingshot arm, late snap of the wrist, fingertip control . . . More than any other athletes except perhaps cyclists, who push their bodies to maximize the torque produced by their machines, quarterbacks must master the complex mechanics of how to move the body through space with balance, control, and power.

Muscles and the bones they are attached to act as levers. To raise the forearm, for instance, the bicep pulls against the elbow, the arm's fulcrum, which magnifies the movement so effectively that the muscle has only to contract slightly to move the forearm several inches.

Individual muscles are organized according to the type and amount of pulling they do, and their architecture is defined by the arrangement of muscle fibers relative to the "force-generating axis"—the direction in which they are pulling. Spindle-shaped fusiform muscles, in which all fibers are the same length and arranged in parallel, are reddish straps that taper at the end and are best for fast and large movements. The fibers in feather-shaped pinnate muscles are angled on both sides of an axis and can deliver more strength than "strap" muscles of the same length. Circular muscles attached to the bony eye socket and to the eyelids open and close the eyes.

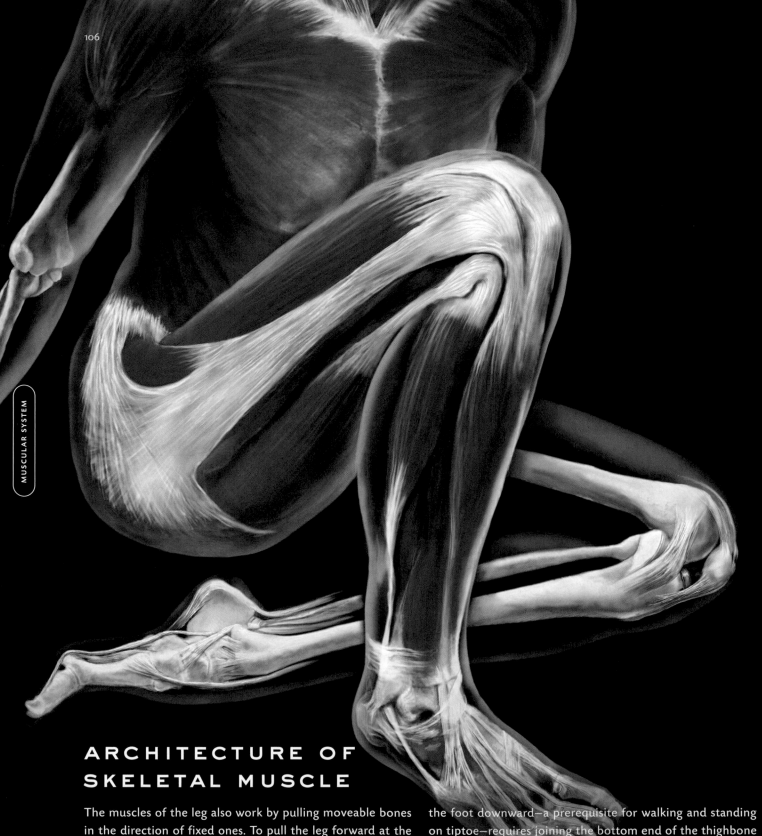

ARCHITECTURE OF SKELETAL MUSCLE

The muscles of the leg also work by pulling moveable bones in the direction of fixed ones. To pull the leg forward at the knee involves connecting the pelvis and thighbone to the shinbone, via a tendon that runs over the kneecap. To bend the foot downward—a prerequisite for walking and standing on tiptoe—requires joining the bottom end of the thighbone to the heel bone via a fleshy muscle in the calf and the strongest tendon in the body, the Achilles.

5

A classic biological example of the structure-function relationship, skeletal muscle is a system with a single purpose—generating force—and it delivers power and velocity by marshaling muscle fibers into a kind of unidirectional motor.

The muscles of the shoulder, for example, exert force for a variety of uses. Those in front lift the arm, pull it forward, rotate it, as well as bend the head forward, and turn and tilt it to one side. Those in the back keep the head upright and bend it in the opposite direction.

Packed in layers, strapped to bones with collagen-rich tendons, shoulder muscles pull the skeletal members of the chest, back, neck, and upper arms across a series of joints to produce both movement and stability. Some remain partially contracted all the time, stiffening the region for upright support.

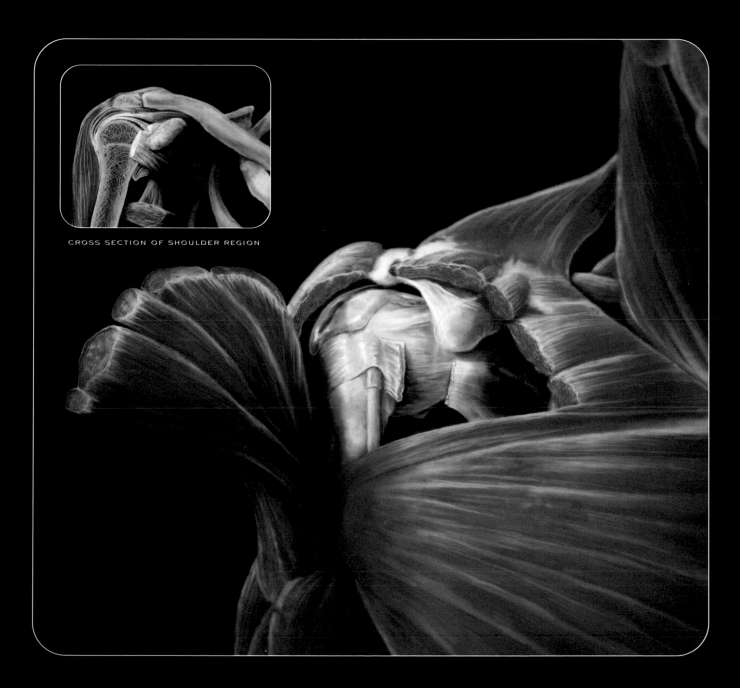

CROSS SECTION OF SHOULDER REGION

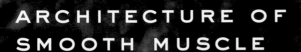

ARCHITECTURE OF SMOOTH MUSCLE

Peristalsis, the mechanism by which smooth muscle—which has no attachment to bone—creates motion, is a "roster system." Tough, ringlike muscles in the gullet rotate tours of duty. Contracting and relaxing in sequence, they push swallowed lumps of food down to the stomach with such force as to keep them down (reversing the process if necessary). Like steel belts in a radial tire, the parallel rings strengthen the whole design while creating a "traveling wave" that pushes against the longitudinal layer of muscle just ahead of it, which in turn relaxes to make space for the next lump.

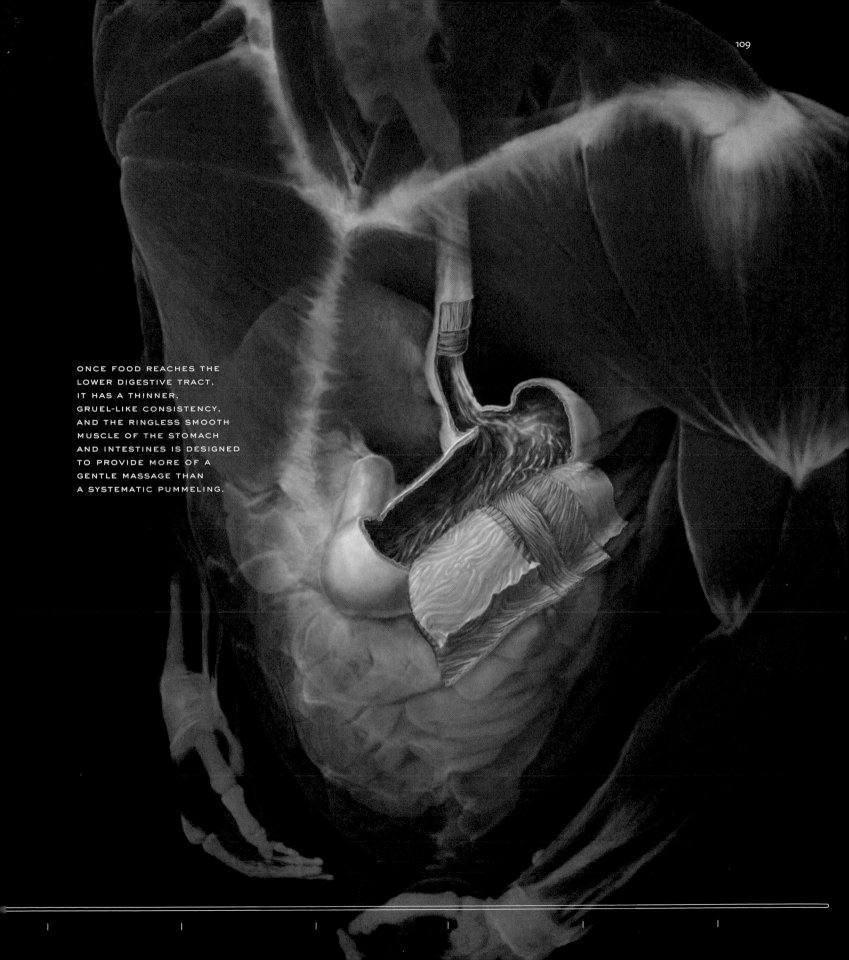

ONCE FOOD REACHES THE
LOWER DIGESTIVE TRACT,
IT HAS A THINNER,
GRUEL-LIKE CONSISTENCY,
AND THE RINGLESS SMOOTH
MUSCLE OF THE STOMACH
AND INTESTINES IS DESIGNED
TO PROVIDE MORE OF A
GENTLE MASSAGE THAN
A SYSTEMATIC PUMMELING.

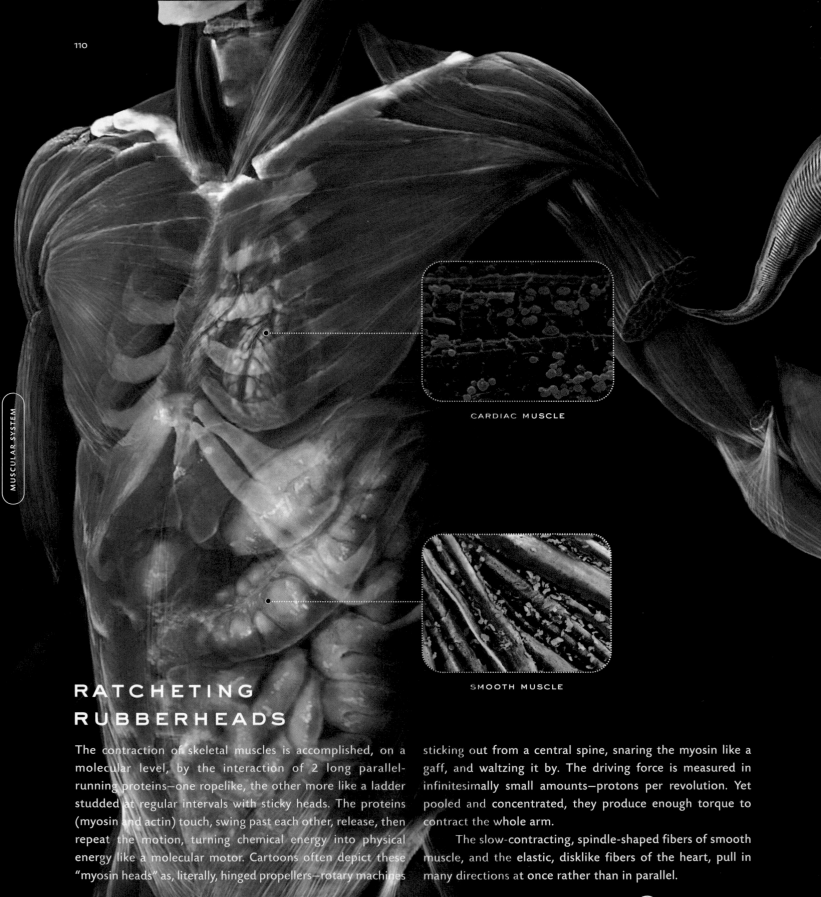

CARDIAC MUSCLE

SMOOTH MUSCLE

RATCHETING RUBBERHEADS

The contraction of skeletal muscles is accomplished, on a molecular level, by the interaction of 2 long parallel-running proteins—one ropelike, the other more like a ladder studded at regular intervals with sticky heads. The proteins (myosin and actin) touch, swing past each other, release, then repeat the motion, turning chemical energy into physical energy like a molecular motor. Cartoons often depict these "myosin heads" as, literally, hinged propellers—rotary machines

sticking out from a central spine, snaring the myosin like a gaff, and waltzing it by. The driving force is measured in infinitesimally small amounts—protons per revolution. Yet pooled and concentrated, they produce enough torque to contract the whole arm.

The slow-contracting, spindle-shaped fibers of smooth muscle, and the elastic, disklike fibers of the heart, pull in many directions at once rather than in parallel.

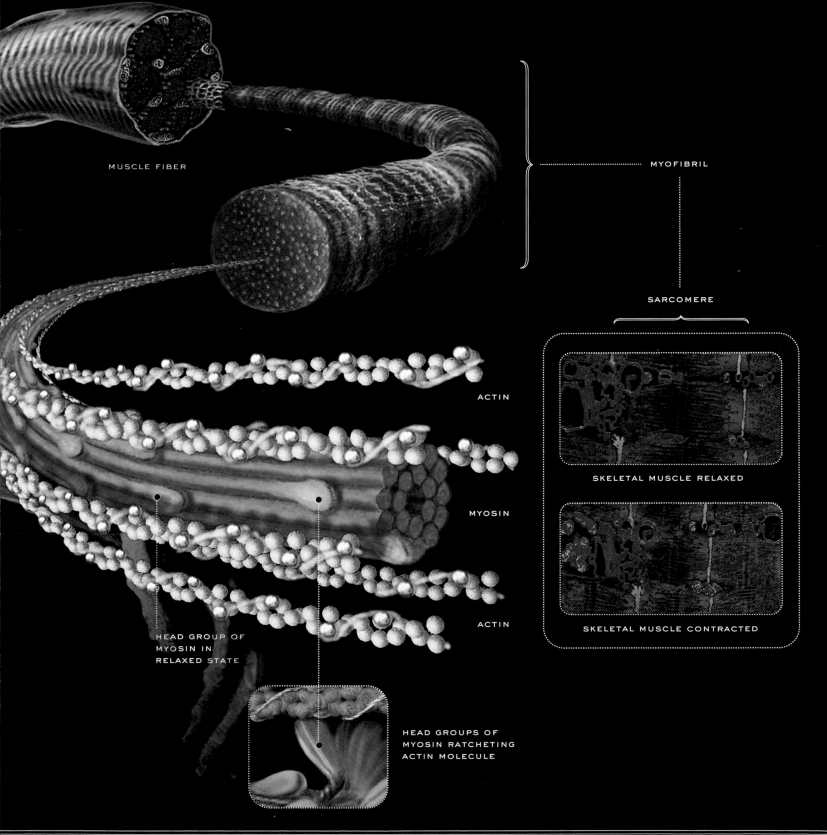

MUSCLE FIBER

MYOFIBRIL

SARCOMERE

ACTIN

MYOSIN

SKELETAL MUSCLE RELAXED

ACTIN

SKELETAL MUSCLE CONTRACTED

HEAD GROUP OF
MYOSIN IN
RELAXED STATE

HEAD GROUPS OF
MYOSIN RATCHETING
ACTIN MOLECULE

MIRRORED IN NATURE

A single fiber does not make a thread, nor a tree a forest.
—Chinese proverb

The bundling of microscopic filaments into working structures is a prime example of natural architecture that exceeds the sum of its parts. The fibers in muscles not only connect but

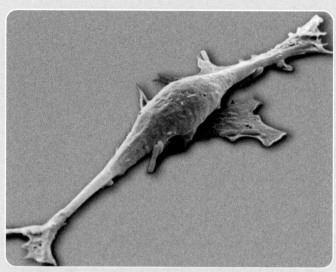

SMOOTH MUSCLE

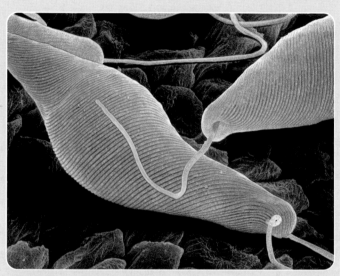

PROTIST

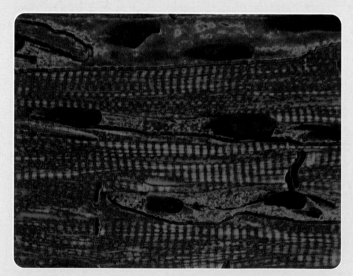

CARDIAC MUSCLE FIBERS

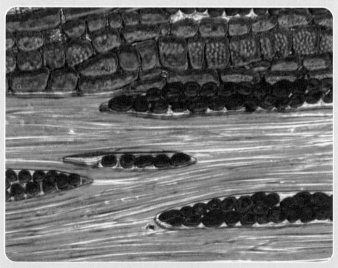

TRANSVERSE CROSS SECTION OF ASH WOOD

empower, bestowing physical strength and also character—"eternal toughness and sinewy fiber," as someone once said of Ulysses S. Grant. It was Achilles whose vulnerable heel exposed

how even the toughest and most resilient fibrous structures can overstretch, wear out and snap, or be pierced and cut, and thus become disabled.

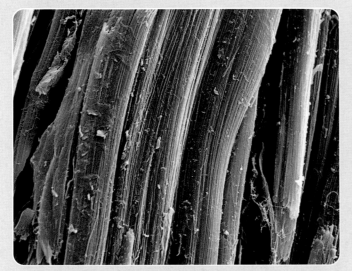

TENDONS OF THE FOOT

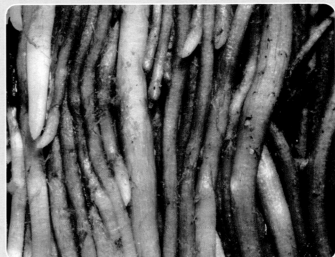

CYPRESS ROOTS

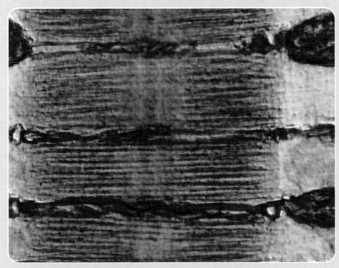

STRIATED MUSCLE FIBERS

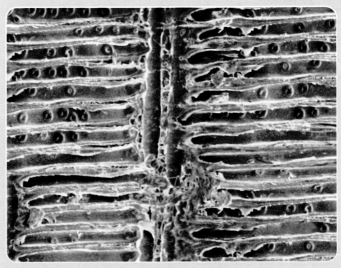

XYLEM OF PLANT

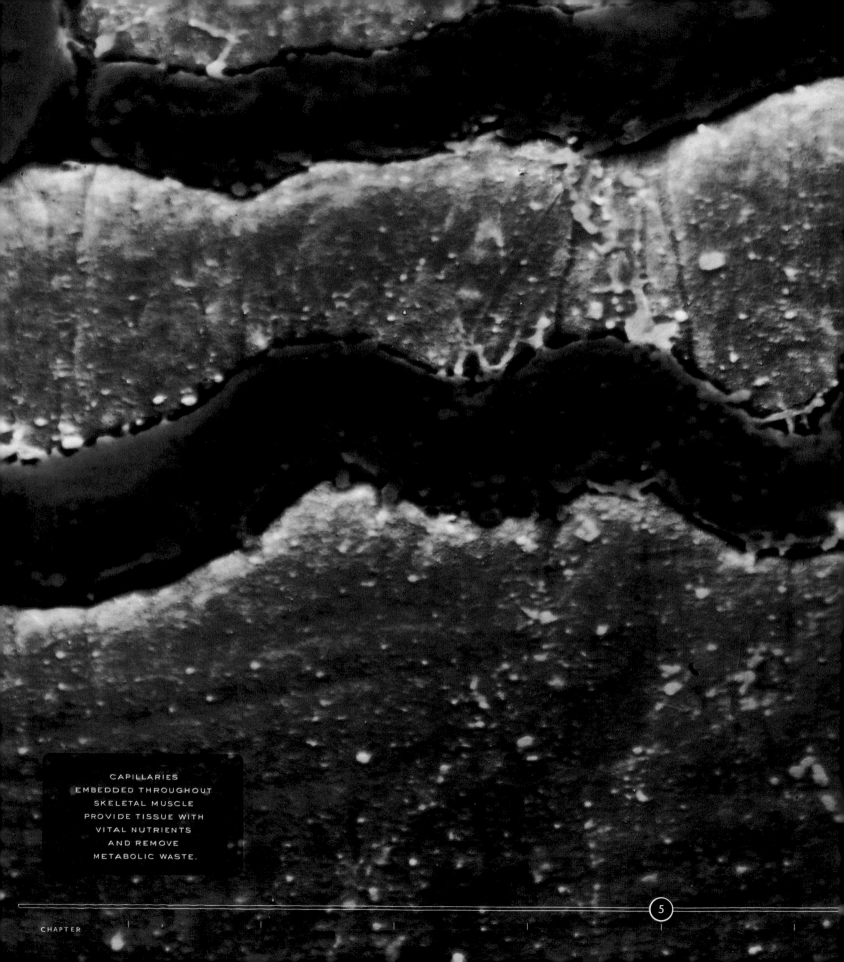

CAPILLARIES
EMBEDDED THROUGHOUT
SKELETAL MUSCLE
PROVIDE TISSUE WITH
VITAL NUTRIENTS
AND REMOVE
METABOLIC WASTE.

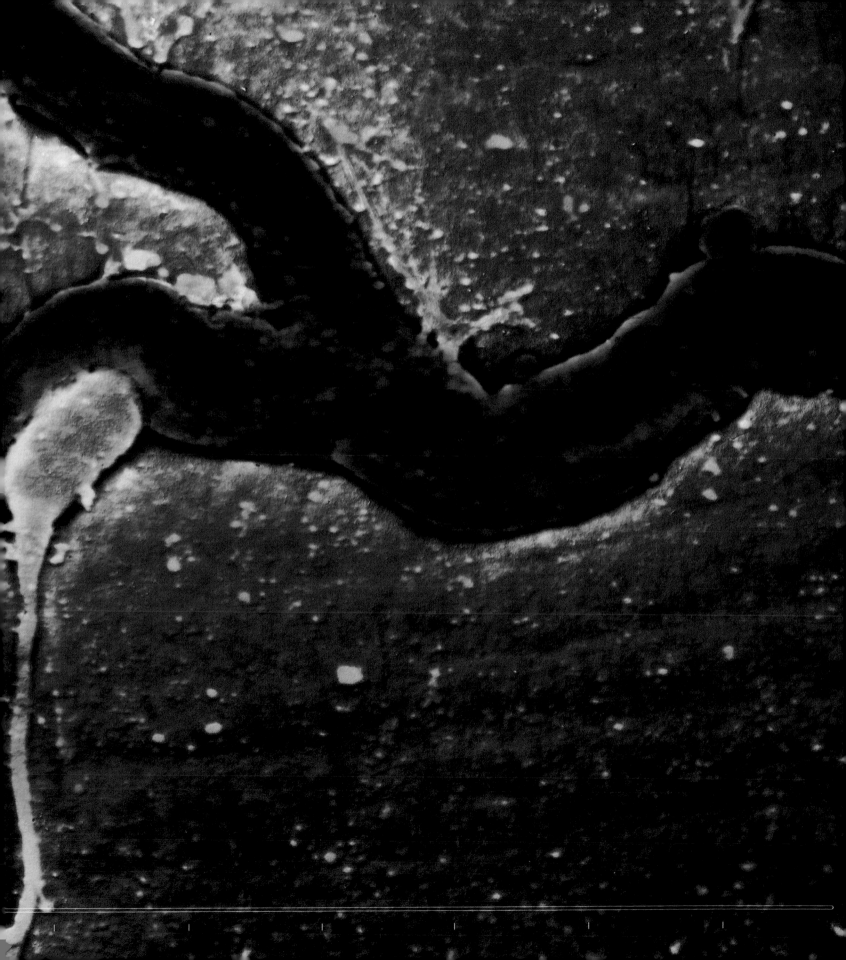

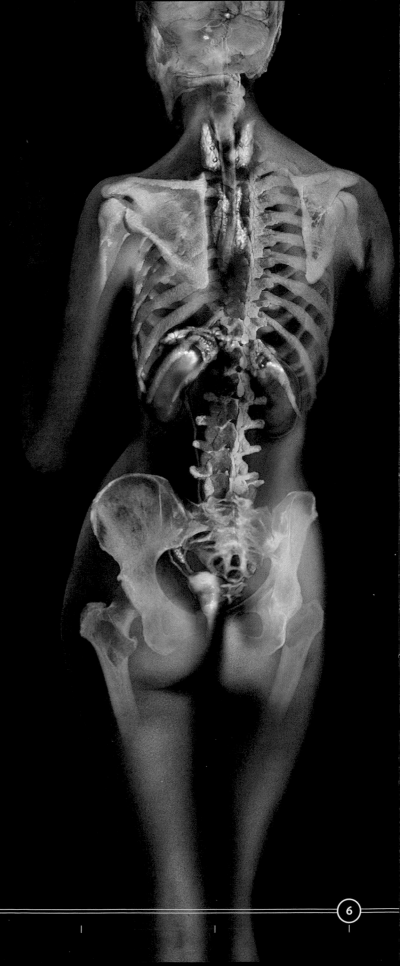

control– chemical

(endocrine system)

In his influential 1932 book *The Wisdom of the Body*, Harvard physiologist Walter Cannon coined the term *homeostasis*, from the Greek words for "same" and "steady." A homeostatic system—be it the earth's environment, the world oil market, a car and driver, a society, a person, or a cell—maintains its structure and activities by means of internal control devices. That is, self-regulation. Homeostasis explains how our bodies keep a constant temperature despite 100-degree swings in the weather, how a baby's sucking stimulates a breast to release milk, how we all aren't diabetic, disabled by too much or too little blood sugar. It explains how we can survive in an ever-changing world. "Not being able to control events, I

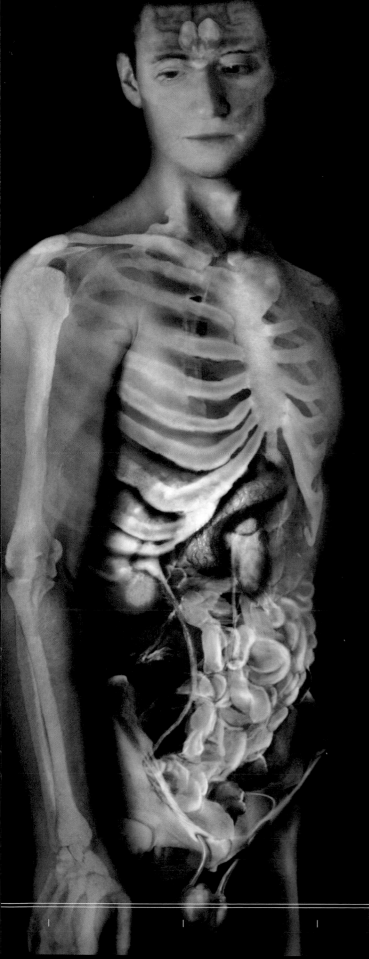

control myself," the Renaissance essayist Michel de Montaigne wrote, "and I adapt myself to them, if they do not adapt themselves to me."

Like the autonomic nervous system, which regulates bodily activity through circular *feedback loops* (another term of Cannon's; his "wisdom" in a nutshell), the far-flung hormone-producing glands of the endocrine system control the body's toweringly complex chemical enterprise through an elaborate hierarchy of signals and counter-signals—a cyclical system of stimulus, monitoring, and response. Unlike the nervous system, the endocrine mechanisms (and the information they carry) are chemicals, which are transported through the blood, thereby requiring a more diffuse architecture.

COMMAND AND CONTROL

Hormones, from the Greek word for "excite" or "spur on," are body chemicals that arouse and dictate the behavior of other body chemicals—molecular dominatrixes. Some of their activity is targeted and some is broadcast (some are like phone calls across town, others like spam mail on the Web), which influences the size, location, and organization of the tissues that produce them.

In addition to homeostasis, hormones also control reproduction, metabolism, behavior, growth, and development— a staggering number of chemical processes each second. Secretory glands grow larger and more productive with age; except, notably, the thymus, a soft, flattened, pinkish-gray organ perched illustriously in front of the heart in infants.

The seat of the immune system, the thymus takes up white cells from the blood and using hormones that it produces, converts them into T cells ("T" for thymus), sentinels that locate, identify, and destroy invaders. The thymus at birth is the size of a fist, in children the size of an orange. But once the immune system is set up around puberty, it shuts down and shrinks significantly. In 2002, Australian immunologists began attempts to "regrow" the gland back to full size, in order to churn out new T cells in patients whose immunities had been destroyed.

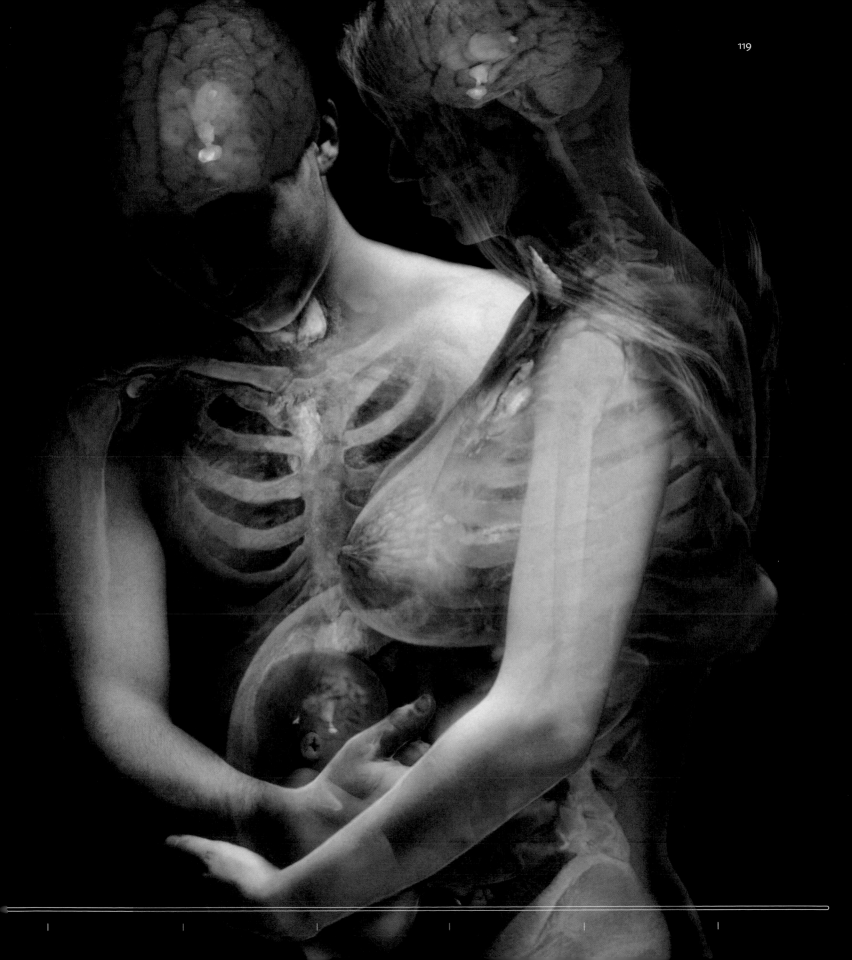

Establishing a flow chart of the body's chemical messaging system has been likened to memorizing the schedules of all the trains, buses, and planes serving New York City. Ten or so major glands and a host of minor ones produce more than 200 hormones and hormonelike substances, each with a specific list of target tissues or "stops," many of them other endocrine organs. As the molecules cascade through the blood, their timetables are maintained by overlapping traffic control systems, each with an array of built-in sensors, monitoring devices, and feedback loops.

The primary centers are located in the head and neck, where they are closely allied with the central nervous system. At the helm is the hypothalamus, the so-called "King of Glands,"

which produces some hormones but most notably connects endocrine function to the brain. A few inches away, the thyroid gland, a blood rich, butterfly-shaped organ in the front of the throat, governs metabolism, including heart rate and energy use, by releasing the hormone thyroxine. When the hypothalamus, which monitors thyroxine concentrations in the blood, senses low levels, it discharges a chemical signal to the neighboring pituitary gland, which in turn releases thyroid stimulating hormone (TSH), which spurs the production of more thyroxine. The parathyroids are 4 small, paired glands that work with the thyroid, drawing calcium from the bones, where it's stored, into the blood for use in activating muscles.

THE KING OF GLANDS
AND HIS COURT

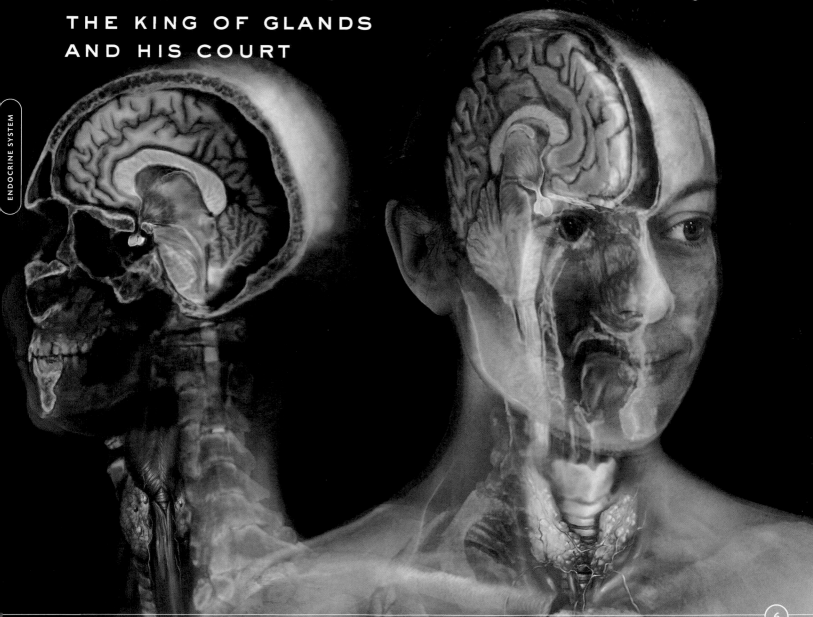

Males, as Natalie Angier writes, were "the hapless recipients of the first experiments in endocrinology . . . Men were castrated to render them trustworthy." The ancients observed that gelding the testicles made men more manageable and less libidinous, and for centuries promising, preadolescent sopranos were castrated to prevent their vocal cords from thickening, thereby lowering their pitch. Halting the flood of androgens (hormones that spur male sex characteristics) before it started, parents helped produce in their sons a magnificent (and androgynous, and potentially lucrative) vocal instrument: man-sized lungs bellowing through what was essentially a woman's voice box.

Sex differences due to hormonal and physical changes peak at puberty, but distinctions arise before that. In both boys and girls, starting before age 8, rising levels of androgens produced in the adrenal glands may set off premature biochemical surges. More common in girls, these include the precocious sprouting of pubic hair, glandular odors, and acne. With the onset of sex hormone secretion by the gonads, sexual development and reproductive function begin. Although men and women both produce male and female hormones, the effects tend to be gender-specific. Increased testosterone levels have been connected with aggression and social dominance, while fluctuating estrogen levels correlate with mood swings.

In women, the primary source of chemical messengers that sexualize the body—causing pubic hair to grow, fat to gather on the breasts and hips ("gynoid" distribution), the pelvis to widen, and menstruation to start—are the almond-shaped ovaries. These hormones (estrogen steroids) help govern the reproductive cycle. For instance, estradiol, the principle female hormone of the childbearing years, causes the lining of the vagina to become "cornified"—its cells lengthen into shapes resembling ears of corn—during the part of the cycle when the egg is prepared for ovulation. This matures and thickens the vaginal lining, priming it for sexual contact.

MAN

WOMAN

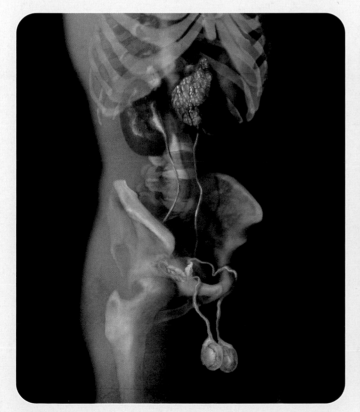

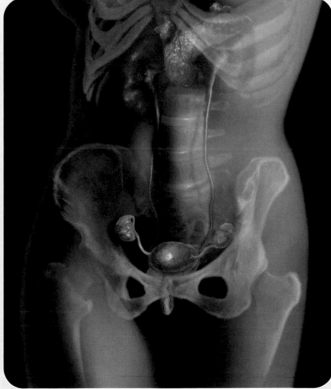

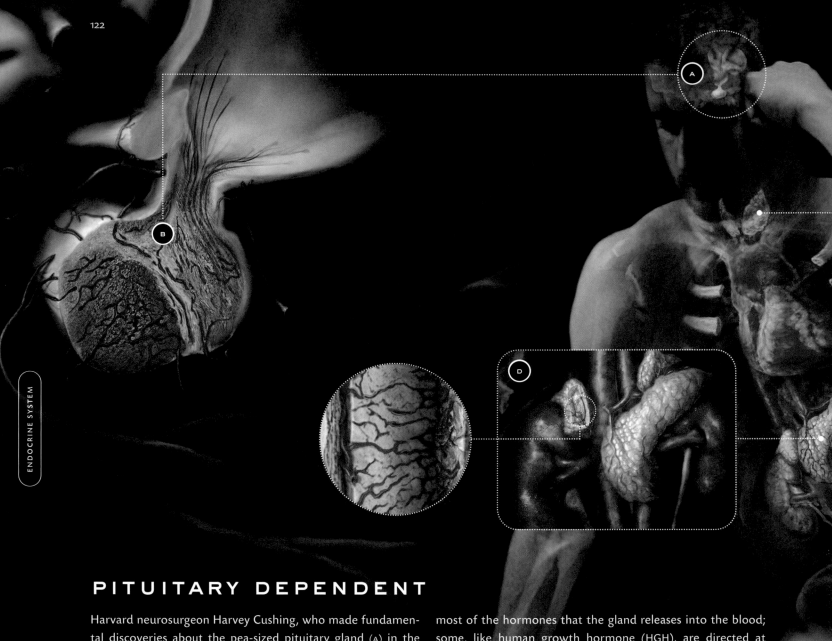

PITUITARY DEPENDENT

Harvard neurosurgeon Harvey Cushing, who made fundamental discoveries about the pea-sized pituitary gland (A) in the decade before World War I, called it "the conductor of the endocrine orchestra." *Concertmaster* may be more fitting—the hypothalamus is the true conductor, interpreting the score, directing the performance. But the relationship between the pituitary's output of 9 major hormones and a range of bodily processes—metabolism, reproduction, breast development, birth, growth, and repair, plus the production of milk, urine, and steroids—still evokes rhapsodic comparisons. "Hormones," Angier notes, "have a music to them, a molecular lyricism."

Attached to the hypothalamus by a short stalk, the pituitary hangs from the base of the brain and has 2 lobes (B). The larger front lobe contains endocrine cells and produces most of the hormones that the gland releases into the blood; some, like human growth hormone (HGH), are directed at increasing the functioning of targeted glands and tissues; others, such as thyroid stimulating hormone (TSH), are aimed at triggering the secretion of other hormones like thyroxine from the thyroid gland (C). The rear lobe is composed mainly of nerve fibers originating in the hypothalamus, and stores the 2 hormones that it releases through a process known as neurosecretion. (Oxytocin, which triggers contractions in the uterus and stimulates the release of breast milk, is one of these, although its function in men remains unclear.)

The hormone ACTH signals the adrenals (D) to produce steroid hormones, including those that help regulate the level of salts and water in the blood.

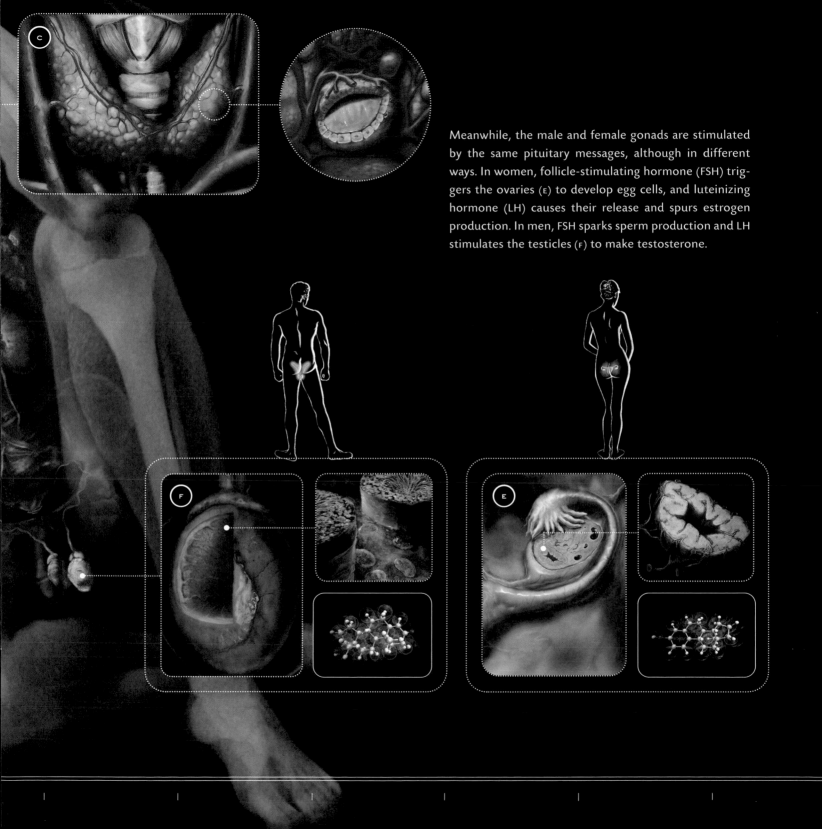

Meanwhile, the male and female gonads are stimulated by the same pituitary messages, although in different ways. In women, follicle-stimulating hormone (FSH) triggers the ovaries (ε) to develop egg cells, and luteinizing hormone (LH) causes their release and spurs estrogen production. In men, FSH sparks sperm production and LH stimulates the testicles (F) to make testosterone.

Running the body, like the maintenance of any homeostatic system, involves regular surveillance and precisely timed and aimed chemical releases. An archipelago of outlying detachments—outposts—infuses the blood with key hormones that control specific daily, even hourly, functions. Tucked away under the brain, the pineal gland (A) secretes melatonin, which regulates body rhythms such as sleeping and waking. The pea-sized parathyroids (B) produce parathormone, helping to adjust blood calcium levels. The thymus (C) secretes hormones which regulate T cell maturation, proliferation and function; cell clusters in the pancreas, the islets of Langerhans (D), make insulin and glucagons which regulate blood glucose; and the kidneys (E) secrete both erythropoietin, which stimulates the production of red blood cells, and renin, which helps control blood pressure. Since all of these products (except T cells) can be synthesized in the lab, many of the diseases caused by their absence are now controlled by replacement therapy.

PITUITARY
NONDEPENDENT

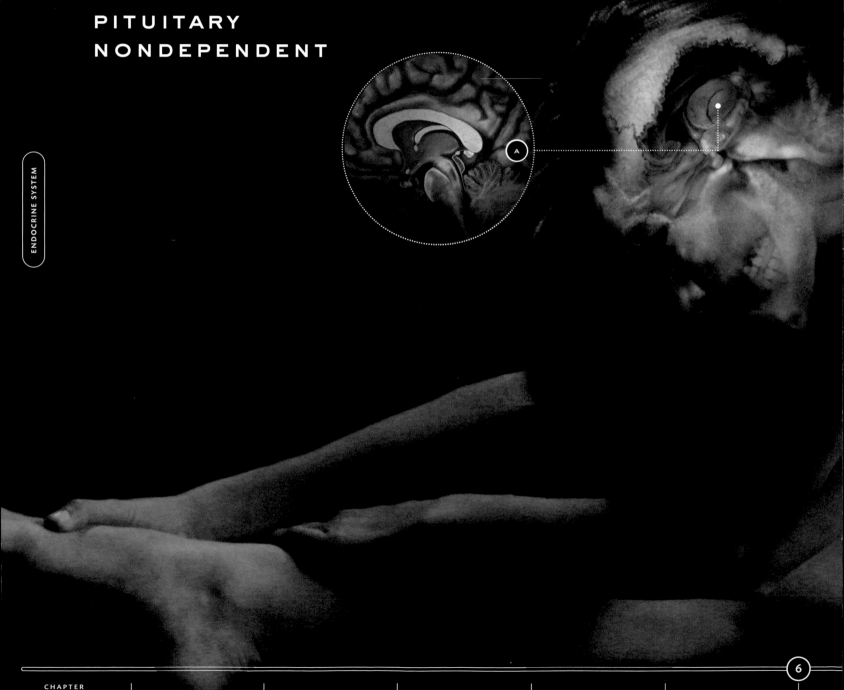

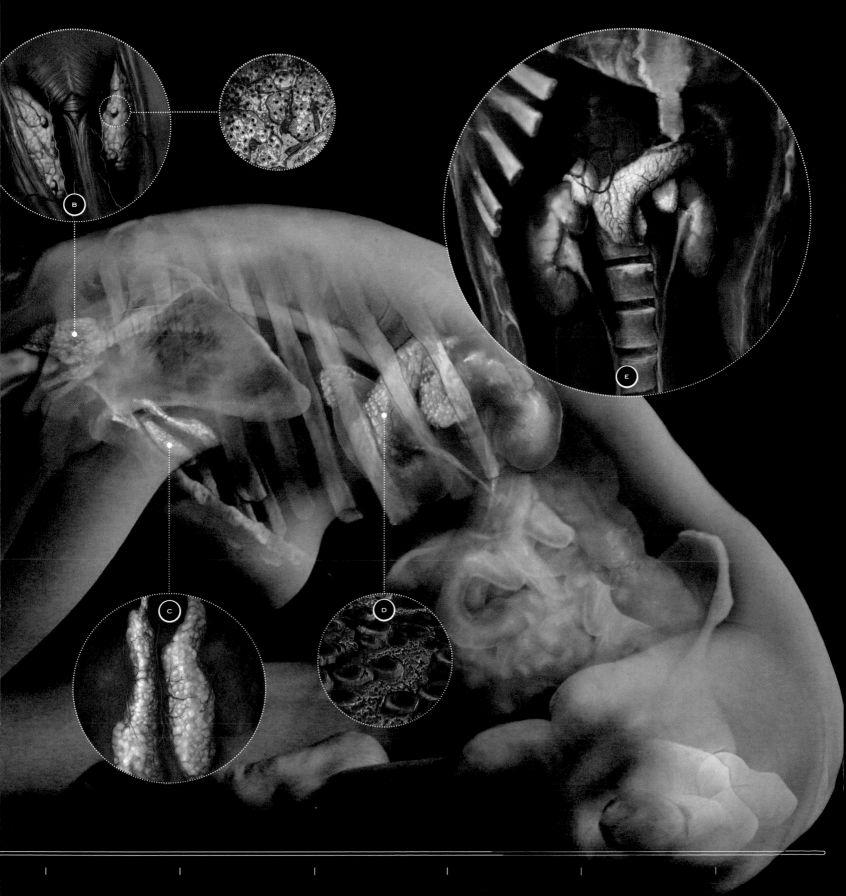

MIRRORED IN NATURE

It's the business of endocrine tissues to secrete complex chemicals, and so their basic structures are optimized for making and transporting large molecules. Like the organelles in green plants that make and store food, spherical sacs fill the thyroid gland; the sacs contain chemicals used to synthesize the primary hormones. Hormones in the pituitary gland target specific tissues, organs,

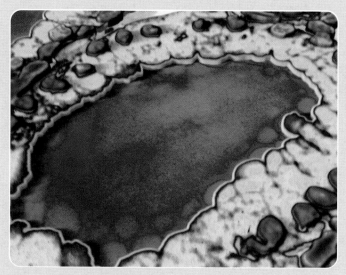

FOLLICULAR CELLS OF A THYROID GLAND

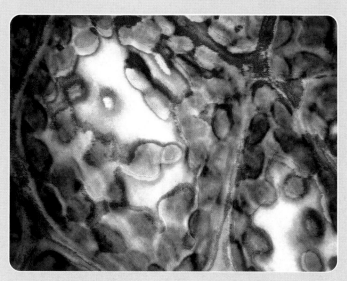

CHLOROPLASTS IN PLANT

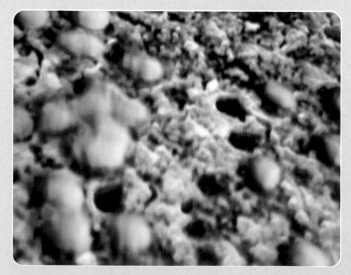

CELLS OF THE PITUITARY GLAND

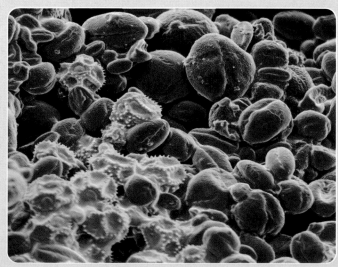

POLLEN GRAINS

and cells much the same way that pollen granules target the reproductive cells of another plant to form seeds, and the tightly coiled tubules of the testicles share the radial symmetry of marine invertebrates. The water-storing cells of a spinach leaf function much like pancreatic cells, which store digestive and hormonal products.

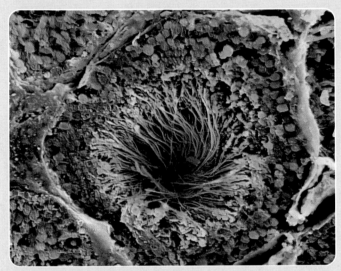

TUBULES IN THE TESTES

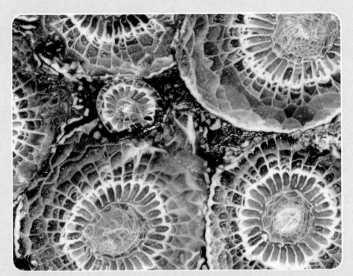

CORAL POLYPS

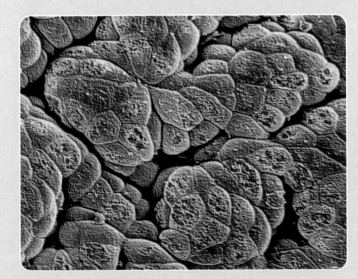

CELLS OF THE PANCREAS

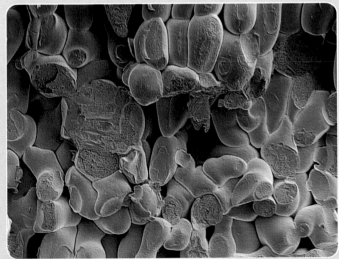

CELLS OF A SPINACH LEAF

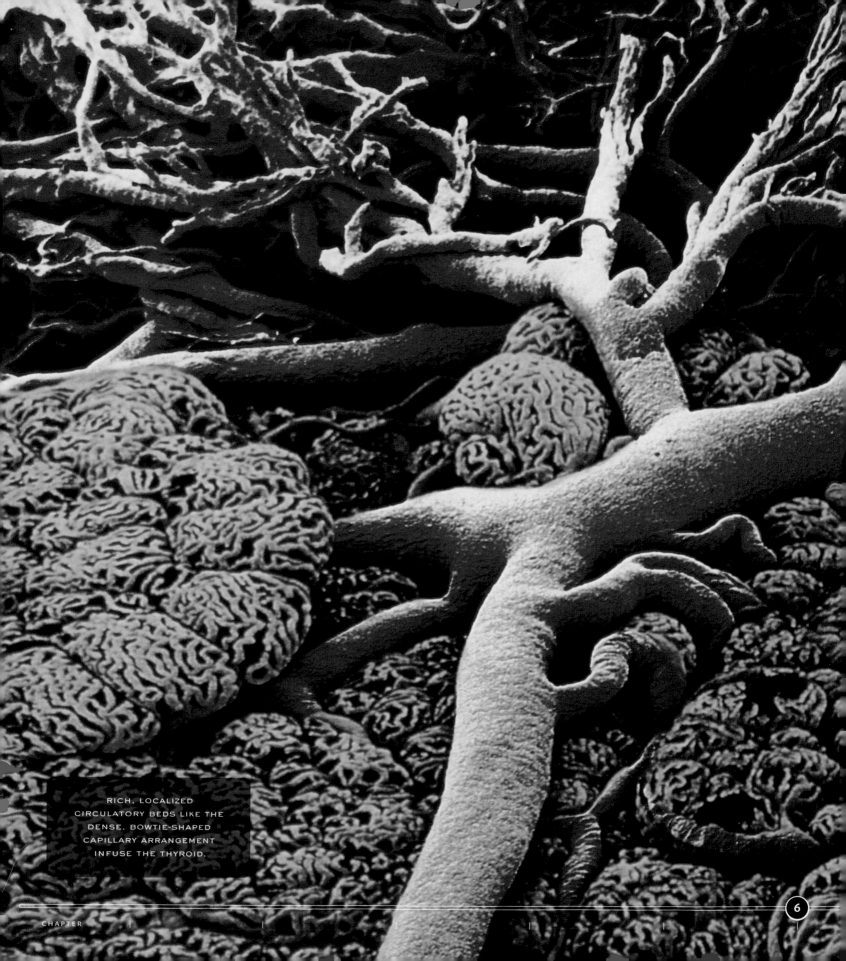

RICH, LOCALIZED
CIRCULATORY BEDS LIKE THE
DENSE, BOWTIE-SHAPED
CAPILLARY ARRANGEMENT
INFUSE THE THYROID.

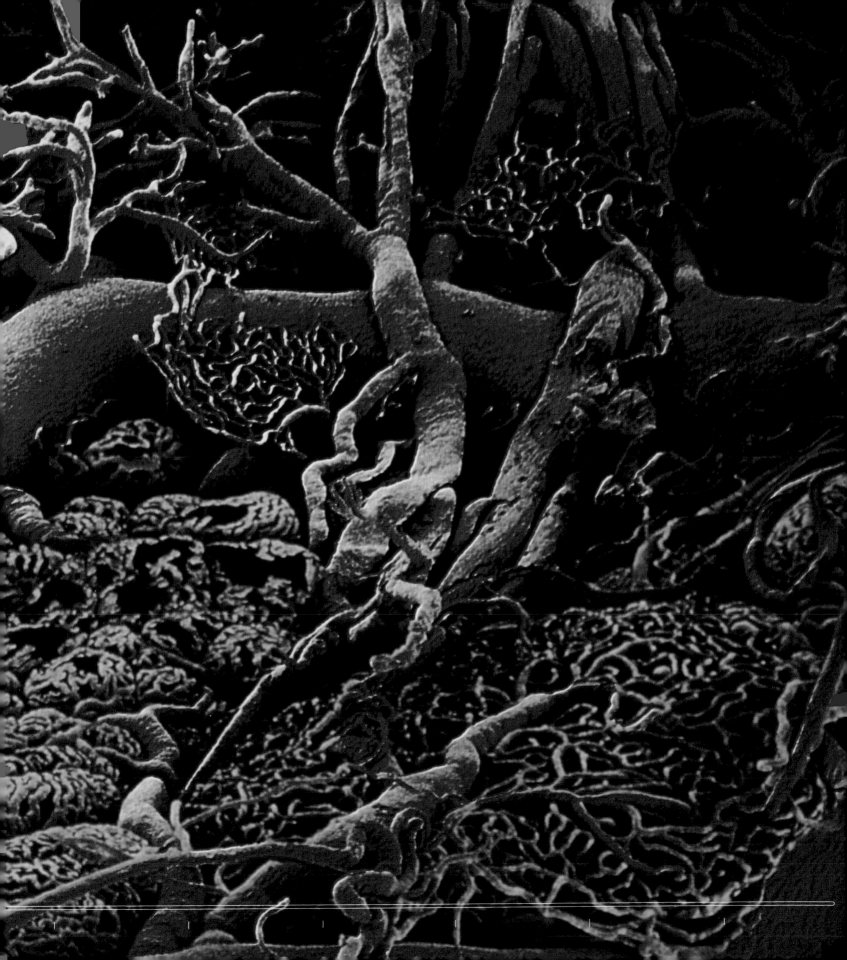

heat circulation

(cardiovascular system)

Though the heart is, mechanically speaking, a pump, and the circulatory system a network of pipes through which liquid tissue flows, physiologists and poets since Aristotle have marveled most at the system's motive (and emotive) power—its *heat* The heart contracts 70- to 80 times each minute (about 100,000 times a day) and expands *on its own steam*, delivering life-sustaining oxygen and nutrients through a system of tubes that, laid end to end, would circle the world 3 to 4 times. Over the course of a 70-year lifetime it will beat 2.5 billion times, pumping approximately 1 million barrels of blood. Such an engine is a dynamo: "the

hearthstone and source of innate heat by which the animal is governed," ancient Greek physician Galen called it.

It is also the organ, along with the brain and senses, most sensitized to (and expressive of) love and beauty, fear and courage. When the Tin Woodman in *The Wizard of Oz* wants "to register emotion, jealousy, devotion, and really feel the part," and to "be kind'a human," he craves a heart. A woman's heart, 25 percent smaller on average than a man's, beats 5 to 8 more times per minute, meaning most women tire sooner than men. Women's hearts also generally last longer. "Who shall measure the heat and violence of the poet's heart when caught and tangled in a woman's body?" Virginia Woolf asked.

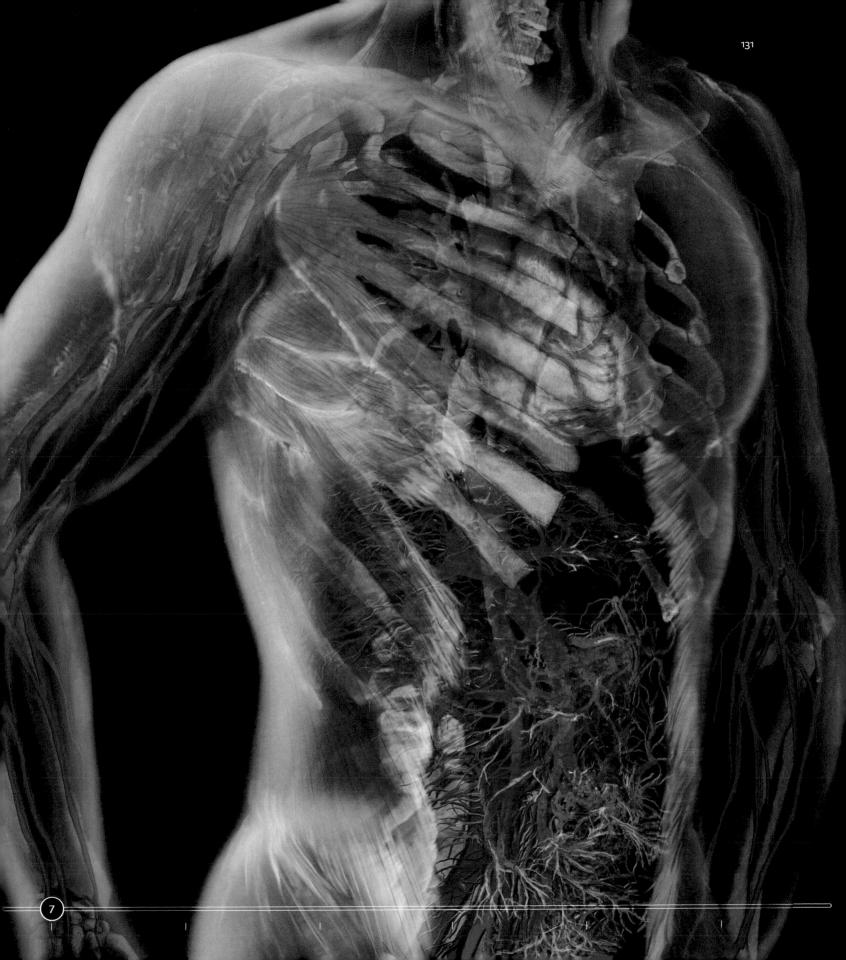

Before birth, the cardiovascular system has no use for the lungs. Gasses are exchanged via the mother, and blood returning from the body to the right atrium (top chamber) is shunted either to the left atrium through a temporary opening called the foramen ovale, an oval-shaped window, or into the thicker-walled right ventricle (bottom chamber). With each pulse, both sides pump blood directly to the body, in parallel, fueling its prodigious growth. Constant high pressure in the deflated lungs stanches any backwash.

In all plumbing systems, liquid rushes from areas of higher to lower pressure, and when our lungs first inflate with air at birth, the heart's mechanics shift. "Pulmonary resistance" drops sharply and more blood gushes from the right atrium into the right ventricle, which pumps it into the lungs through the pulmonary veins. Blood from the lungs then flows into the left atrium, increasing the pressure there.

Altogether, these changes press the tough, elastic wall between the atria to seal the "oval window" shut, thereby completing the separation of the apparatus into 2 halves, left and right. Within days, the major duct diverting blood away from the lungs from the aorta also closes, and the mature heart—in fact 2 pumps in 1—begins to beat.

FIRST, FIXING A HOLE

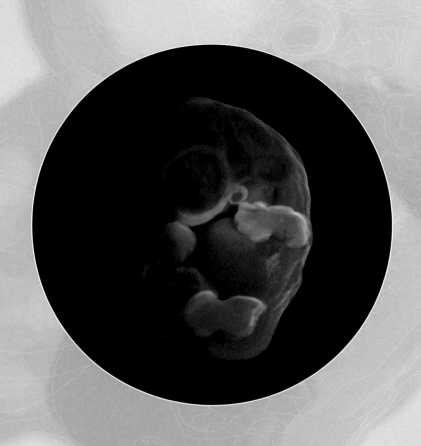

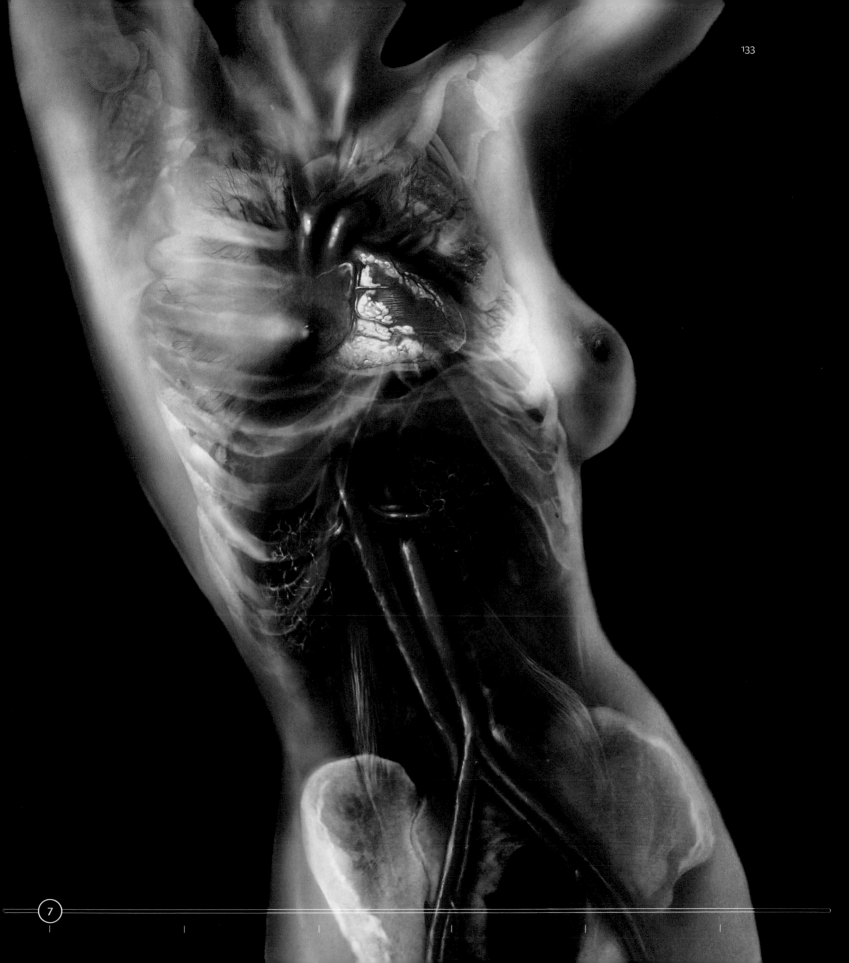

An elegant union of function and form, the heart and blood vessels are designed not just for circulation but *recirculation*—a more complex and dynamic affair. Though continual, the cycle can be said to start when the heart relaxes. The atria fill with blood; valves close to guard against backflow to the lungs and body. Then the atria contract, pushing blood into the ventricles.

The original valves remain closed, but valves between the upper and lower chambers are pushed open. In the third phase, the ventricles contract, sending blood to the lungs and around the body. The surge of blood reopens the first pair of valves while the second pair closes, resetting the apparatus for the next cycle.

THE FULL SYSTEM

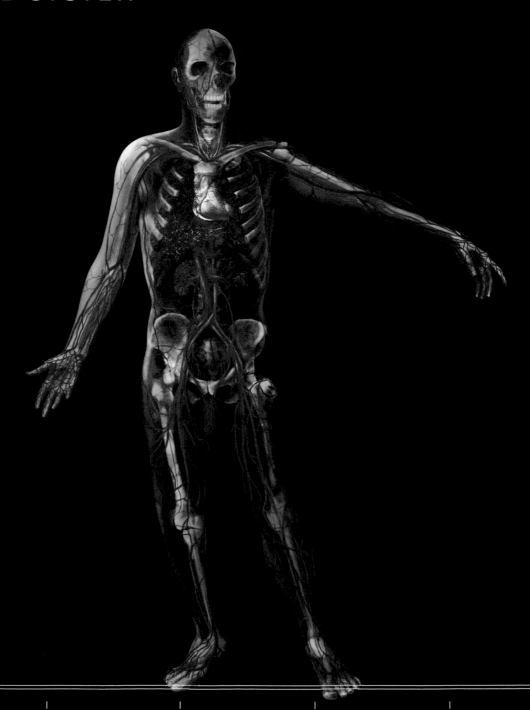

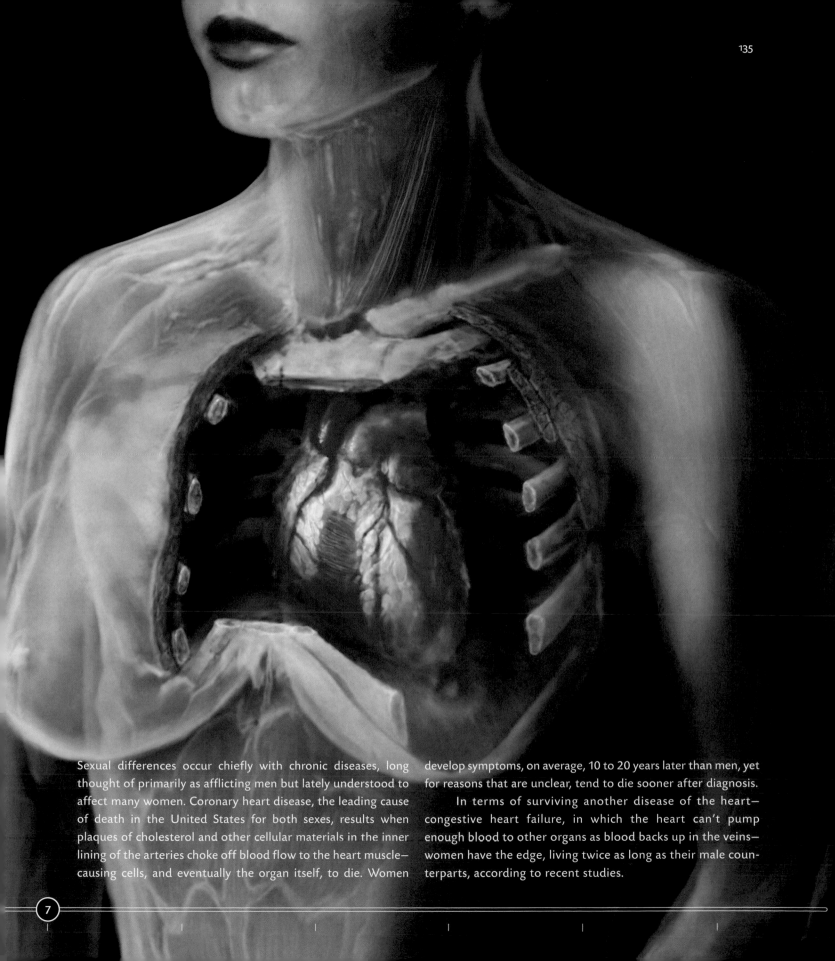

Sexual differences occur chiefly with chronic diseases, long thought of primarily as afflicting men but lately understood to affect many women. Coronary heart disease, the leading cause of death in the United States for both sexes, results when plaques of cholesterol and other cellular materials in the inner lining of the arteries choke off blood flow to the heart muscle—causing cells, and eventually the organ itself, to die. Women develop symptoms, on average, 10 to 20 years later than men, yet for reasons that are unclear, tend to die sooner after diagnosis.

In terms of surviving another disease of the heart—congestive heart failure, in which the heart can't pump enough blood to other organs as blood backs up in the veins—women have the edge, living twice as long as their male counterparts, according to recent studies.

Wrapped around a cloverleaf of 4 tough fibrous rings, or cuffs, to which the 4 heart valves and cardiac muscle are affixed, the heart generates nonstop power by contracting rhythmically . . . over and over . . . without tiring . . . in order to squirt blood along a figure-8 path—first through the lungs to pick up oxygen, then around the body to deliver it.

A natural pacemaker called the sinoatrial (SA) node triggers the cycle. Embedded in the wall of the upper right atrium, it emits regular electrical pulses that race along nervelike cables through the atria, inducing them to contract. The signals pause slightly at a second node before branching left and right, subdividing into a network of modified muscle fibers in the walls of the ventricles. As each burst of electricity reaches the muscle fibers, they contract in turn.

FLOW MECHANICS

(We've Got Rhythm)

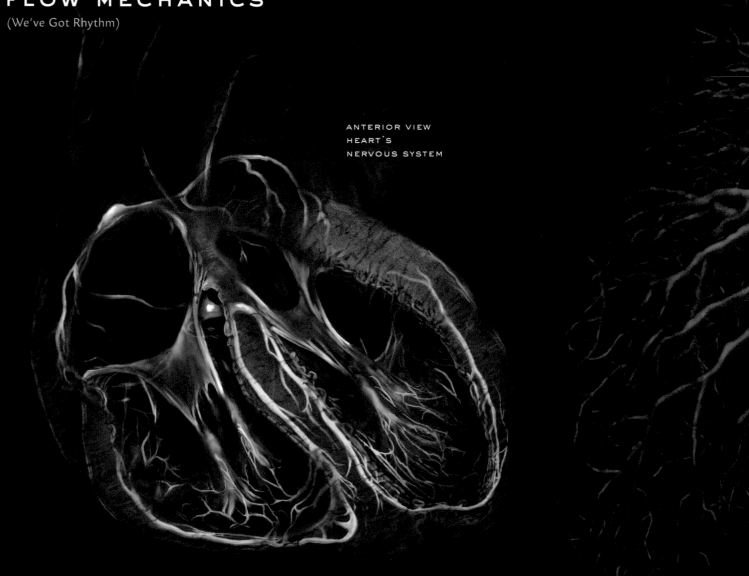

ANTERIOR VIEW
HEART'S
NERVOUS SYSTEM

Importantly, the wiring is designed so that the contractions start at the base of the heart and work their way upward, like a crowd "wave" at a ball game. This ensures that blood is ejected into the major vessels instead of pooling in the bottom of the pointed chambers. Such ceaseless activity exacts a price, in oxygen. Only the brain requires more, and so the heart muscle has its own separate network of blood vessels—the coronary system.

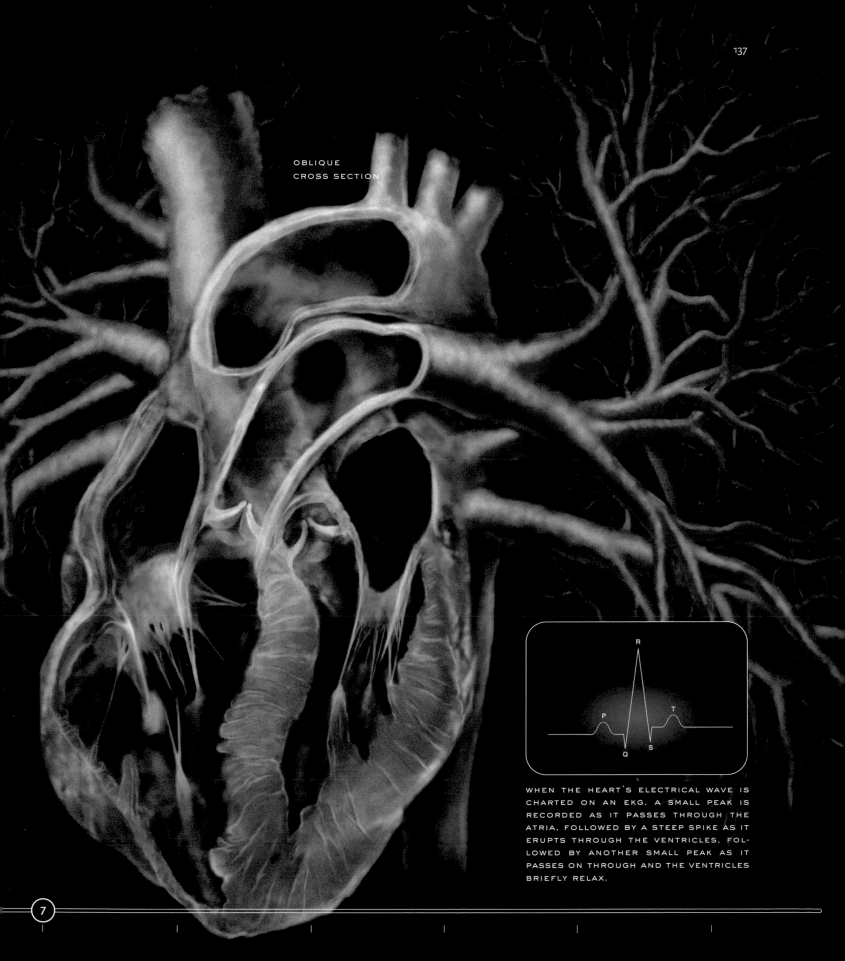

OBLIQUE
CROSS SECTION

WHEN THE HEART'S ELECTRICAL WAVE IS
CHARTED ON AN EKG, A SMALL PEAK IS
RECORDED AS IT PASSES THROUGH THE
ATRIA, FOLLOWED BY A STEEP SPIKE AS IT
ERUPTS THROUGH THE VENTRICLES, FOL-
LOWED BY ANOTHER SMALL PEAK AS IT
PASSES ON THROUGH AND THE VENTRICLES
BRIEFLY RELAX.

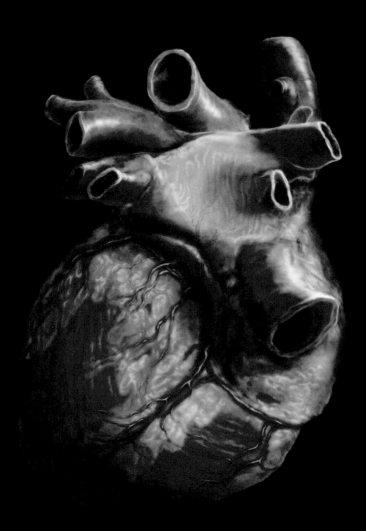

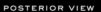

POSTERIOR VIEW

REDUNDANCY AND CONCURRENCE

Beneath the surface of our skin, through which we can often see veins and arteries in our legs, arms, and wrists, lie roughly (depending on body size) 60,000 miles of circulatory apparatus. It's hard to believe, but only one mile of the 60,000 miles of these vessels is visible to the naked eye. The remaining 59,999 are too small to be seen by anything else but microscopes and other powerful imaging technologies. The circulatory system covers so much mileage for a very simple reason: millions and millions of cells need to be fed vital nutrients and drained of their waste. The concurrent and seemingly redundant presence of multiple vessels feeding and draining the same tissues is the best way to accomplish this difficult task. Connections are made as we develop, forming networks of vasculature, commonly known as anastomosis, and because of this we have a built-in

PENETRATING TO THE FARTHEST EXTREMITIES, DELICATE ARTERIES AND VEINS IN THE FEET ADAPT THE RATE AND FLOW OF BLOOD TO THE TOES ACCORDING TO CHANGES IN TEMPERATURE. VESSELS RUNNING AT VARIOUS DEPTHS UNDER THE SKIN IN THE LEG HAVE THE LONGEST ROUTE IN THE BODY. LACKING "PUSH" FROM THE HEART, THESE VEINS ARE AIDED BY SURROUNDING LAYERS OF MUSCLE, THAT SQUEEZE BLOOD BACK TO THE HEART AS THEY CONTRACT.

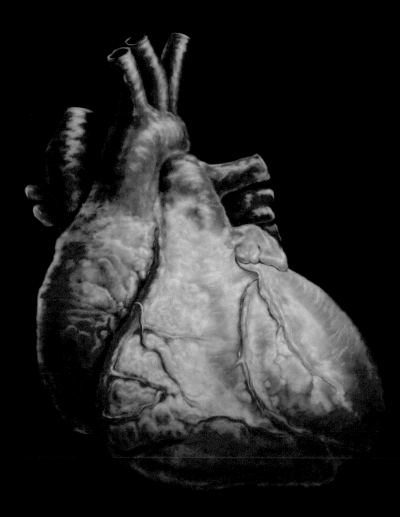

ANTERIOR VIEW

back-up plan. Should any one vessel become damaged or blocked, the body can continue to circulate nutrients to that area.

Viewed at a macroscopic level, the major trunks of arteries lead to their target tissues where they branch continually until they form a capillary bed, exchanging waste with nutrients and then returning to the heart and lungs in the form of veins. In understanding our cardiovascular system, it may be helpful to view each "set" or "pair" of arteries and veins as simple circuits, similar to those in the nervous system where messages are sent and received. Since the same path is needed to transport the blood back to the heart, veins can almost always be found running alongside arteries. Consequently, adjacent veins and arteries commonly share the same anatomical name.

NETWORK OF PIPES

The complex structures of the circulatory system, which not only transports oxygen, nutrients, and waste but also helps regulate the body's water content, temperature, and pH balance, reflect regional differences based on function.

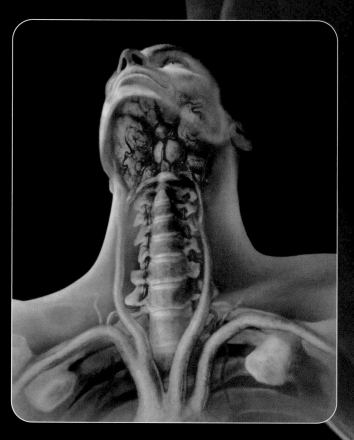

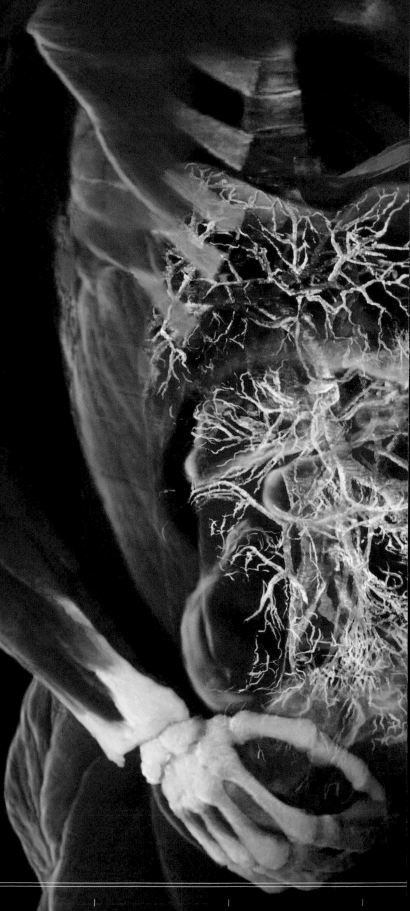

Since the brain uses about one fifth of the oxygen absorbed into the lungs, and brain tissue is at risk of permanent damage after just 5 minutes of blood deprivation, 2 pairs of large vessels—one running through the vertebrae, the other arising from the chest—ensure a generous, constant supply of blood.

In the lower digestive tract, deoxygenated blood from the stomach, spleen, intestines, and pancreas drain into the liver, where nutrients are absorbed and stored and toxins are removed, then returns to the heart and lungs through a large central vein; an independent vascular network (the portal system) with its own smooth-muscle—driven locomotion is required.

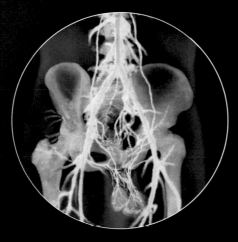

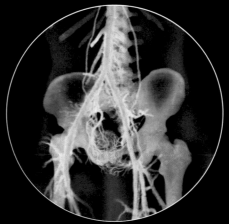

MAN   WOMAN

SEX-BASED FLOW REGIMES

D. H. Lawrence called sex "pure blood consciousness . . . the consciousness of the night." In fact, blood flow to the reproductive organs is vital, involving intricate arrangements of vessels, capillary networks, and, especially, communications between veins and arteries.

Sperm production requires cooler temperatures, which accounts for the location of the testicles outside the body core. The arteries bringing blood to the scrotum are thus narrowly intertwined with the veins that take it away, forming a sophisticated heat exchange mechanism. Rather as with hot and cold water pipes running together, the hot arterial blood loses heat to the cooler venous blood, so blood is cooled as much as 5 to 7 degrees Fahrenheit before it gets to the testes. To produce an erection, blood is needed to engorge 3 cigar-shaped cylinders of spongy mesh that run the length of the penis. As the cylinders

fill with blood, the spongy tissue constricts the veins in their outside walls, compressing them and stopping blood from flowing back out of the penis. With more blood flowing in and less flowing out, the penis becomes—and stays—erect.

In women, periodic disruptions and changes in the body's status quo require vascular structures that can adapt. Chief among these are specialized corkscrew-shaped (spiral) arteries that provide blood to the endometrium, the lining of the uterus. During pregnancy, they flood the placenta with oxygen and nutrients; during menstruation, blood leaks out of their bases, killing endometrial tissue and forcing it to shed. As in men, blood flow is also critical for erotic pleasure, with blood rushing to expand the fibromuscular tube of the vagina, and the mechanism for clitoral engorgement being essentially the same as for erectile tissue in the penis.

WHEN ENGLISH PHYSICIAN WILLIAM HARVEY FIRST
DEMONSTRATED IN THE 1620S THAT BLOOD CIRCULATES
THROUGHOUT THE BODY, HE PREDICTED A NETWORK OF
TINY, THIN-WALLED MICROTUBULES LINKING THE SMALLEST
ARTERIES TO THE SMALLEST VEINS. CAPILLARIES (FROM
THE LATIN FOR "HAIRLIKE") WERE FIRST OBSERVED UNDER
A MICROSCOPE THIRTY YEARS LATER. THE SMALLEST ARE SO
NARROW THAT RED BLOOD CELLS, WHICH MEASURE $^1/_{3,600}$
INCH ACROSS, MUST PASS THROUGH IN SINGLE FILE.

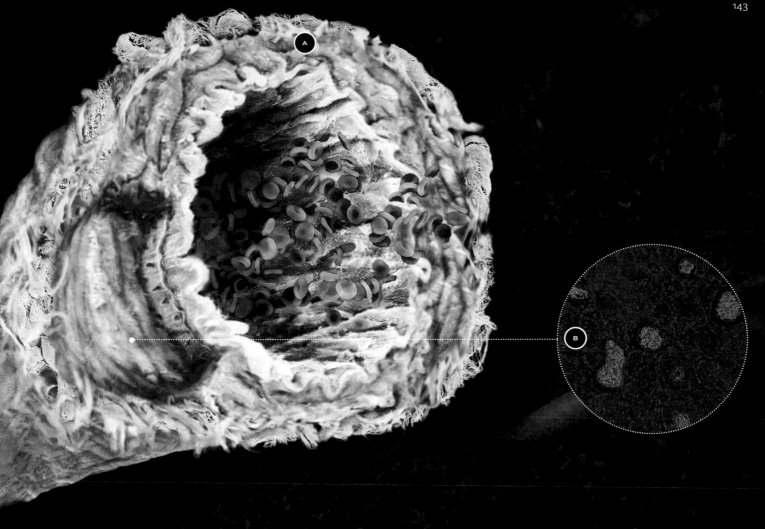

ARTERIES, CAPILLARIES, AND VEINS

Superficially, arteries and veins look alike. Running in parallel, they have about the same thickness. But structurally they differ. Arteries (A), carrying oxygen-rich blood from the heart to the tissues under high pressure, have in their walls a wide middle layer of muscle fibers and elastic tissue, which allows them to expand and recoil as the heart contracts. Smaller arterioles are wrapped in smooth muscle fibers (B) that contract and relax, regulating blood flow and pressure. Veins (C), on the other hand, transport spent blood back to the heart under low pressure. They have thinner walls, making them more susceptible to contractions in surrounding muscles, and a succession of valve flaps to prevent backflow. Moving desultorily through wider lumens (the interior space through which blood flows), venous blood comprises more than $2/3$ of the body's supply at any given time.

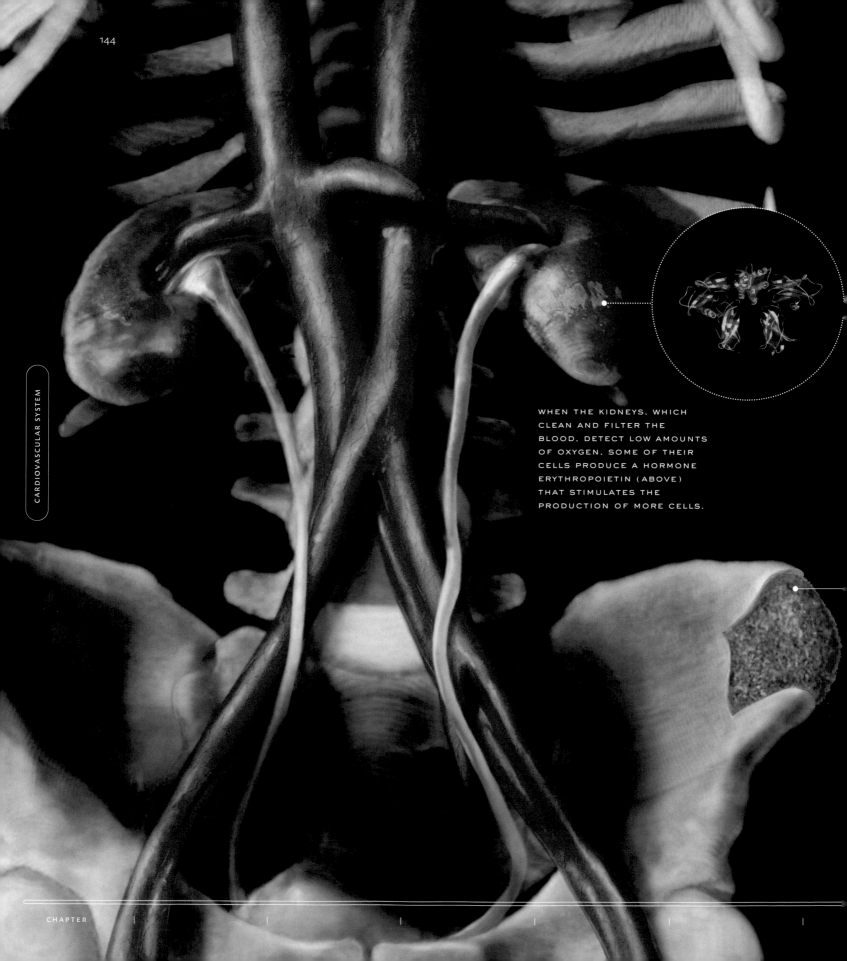

CARDIOVASCULAR SYSTEM

WHEN THE KIDNEYS, WHICH
CLEAN AND FILTER THE
BLOOD, DETECT LOW AMOUNTS
OF OXYGEN, SOME OF THEIR
CELLS PRODUCE A HORMONE
ERYTHROPOIETIN (ABOVE)
THAT STIMULATES THE
PRODUCTION OF MORE CELLS.

Hemoglobin (RIGHT), a large, globe-shaped protein in red blood cells (and the first protein for which the atom-by-atom architecture was solved), represents a perfect marriage of function and form. Each molecule (every cell has about 250 million) consists of 2 pairs of folded chains of atoms, each of which contains a reddish iron atom that, like a submicroscopic magnet, picks up and drops off oxygen atoms. Oxygen in the lungs' air sacs combines with the iron, "catches the wave," then is released downstream in the capillaries, where it's taken up by surrounding cells and used to produce energy.

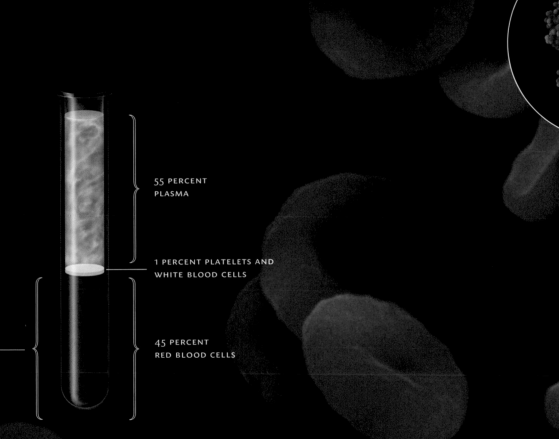

55 PERCENT
PLASMA

1 PERCENT PLATELETS AND
WHITE BLOOD CELLS

45 PERCENT
RED BLOOD CELLS

LIQUID LIFE

Like bone and cartilage, blood can be seen as a connective tissue, a mass of cells imbedded in a framework. However, because its job is mobile, not fixed, its matrix is a liquid—plasma. Suspended in plasma are trillions of blood cells. Dimpled, disk-shaped red blood cells, built to provide a large surface in relation to volume, transport oxygen to tissues. Granular, many-lobed white blood cells, outnumbered by about 700 to 1, comprise a mobile defense force. Platelets, designed to aid in tissue repair, are tiny round or oval cell fragments that congregate around damaged sites in the bloodstream, swelling and sticking to each other to form temporary plugs that can stop leaks.

Red blood cells live only about 3 to 4 months, dying at a rate of about 2 million per second. They're resupplied in equal numbers, however, by the body's red bone marrow, a spongy, colony-spawning matrix inside the bones, such as the pelvis.

MIRRORED IN NATURE

"Go at nightfall to the top of one of the downtown steel giants and you may see how in the image of material man, at once his glory and his menace, is this thing we call a city . . . Thousands of acres of cellular tissue, the city's flesh outspreads layer upon layer, enmeshed by an intricate network of veins and arteries radiating into the gloom, and in them, with muffled, persistent roar, circulating as the blood circulates in your veins, is the almost ceaseless beat of the activity to whose necessities it all conforms."—Frank Lloyd Wright, 1904

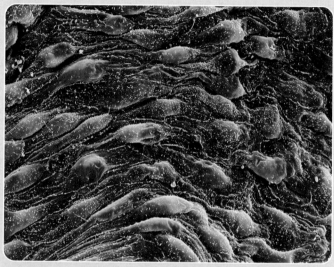

ENDOTHELIUM OF A BLOOD VESSEL

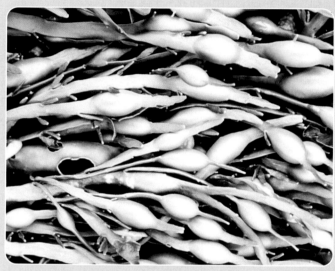

AIR BLADDERS IN SEAWEED

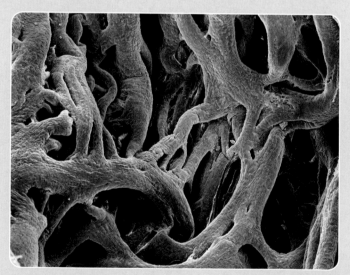

HEART VALVE TENDONS

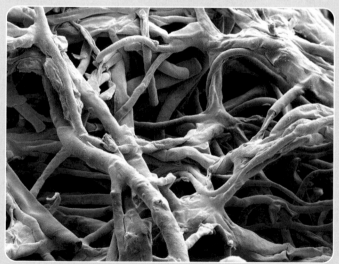

PENICILLIUM

From an architectural standpoint, it's hard to improve on Wright's comparison between "material man" and a pulsing metropolis. The living forms associated with circulation—elastic muscle cells, tubular vessels, and spherical and donut-shaped blood cells— evoke others in nature whose primary job is the movement of living matter around citylike entities that stay up all night.

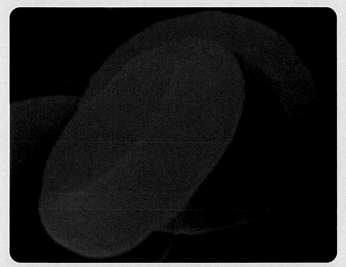

RED BLOOD CELL

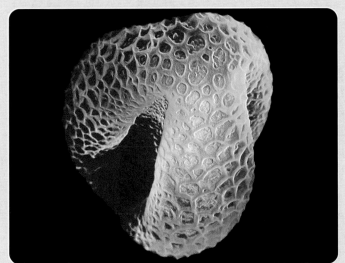

POLLEN

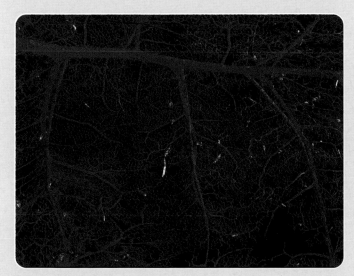

BLOOD VESSELS

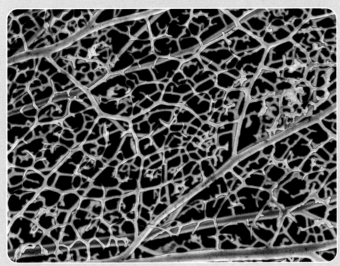

VEINS IN A LEAF

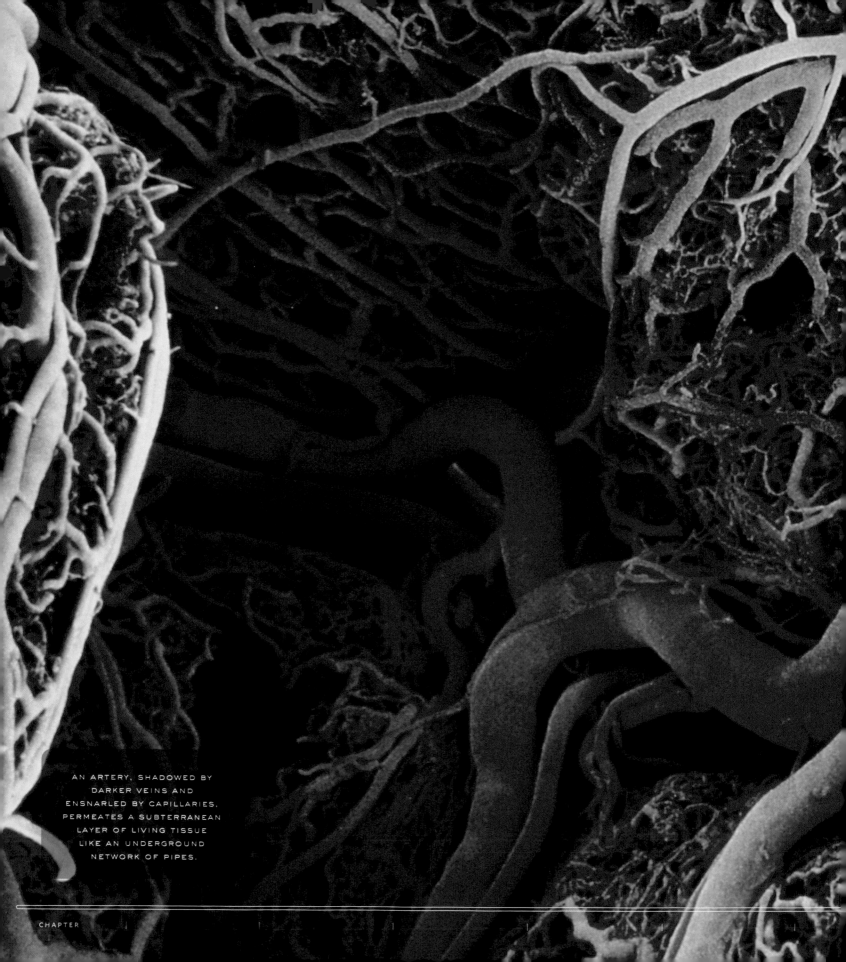

AN ARTERY, SHADOWED BY
DARKER VEINS AND
ENSNARLED BY CAPILLARIES,
PERMEATES A SUBTERRANEAN
LAYER OF LIVING TISSUE
LIKE AN UNDERGROUND
NETWORK OF PIPES.

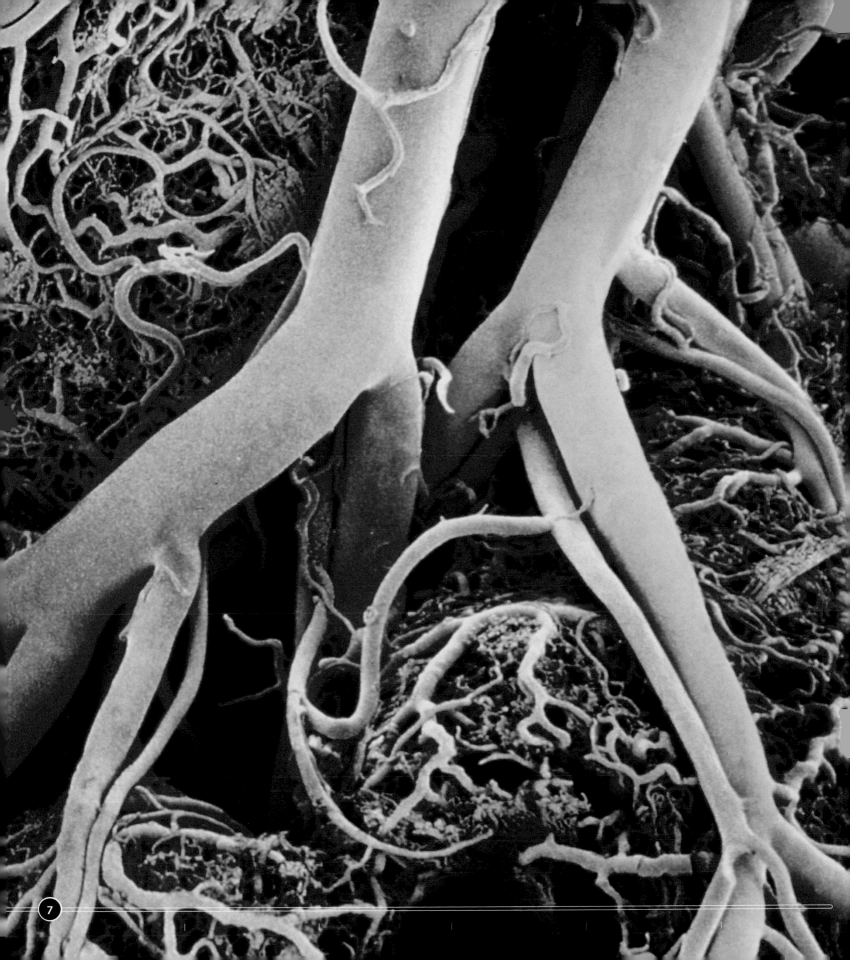

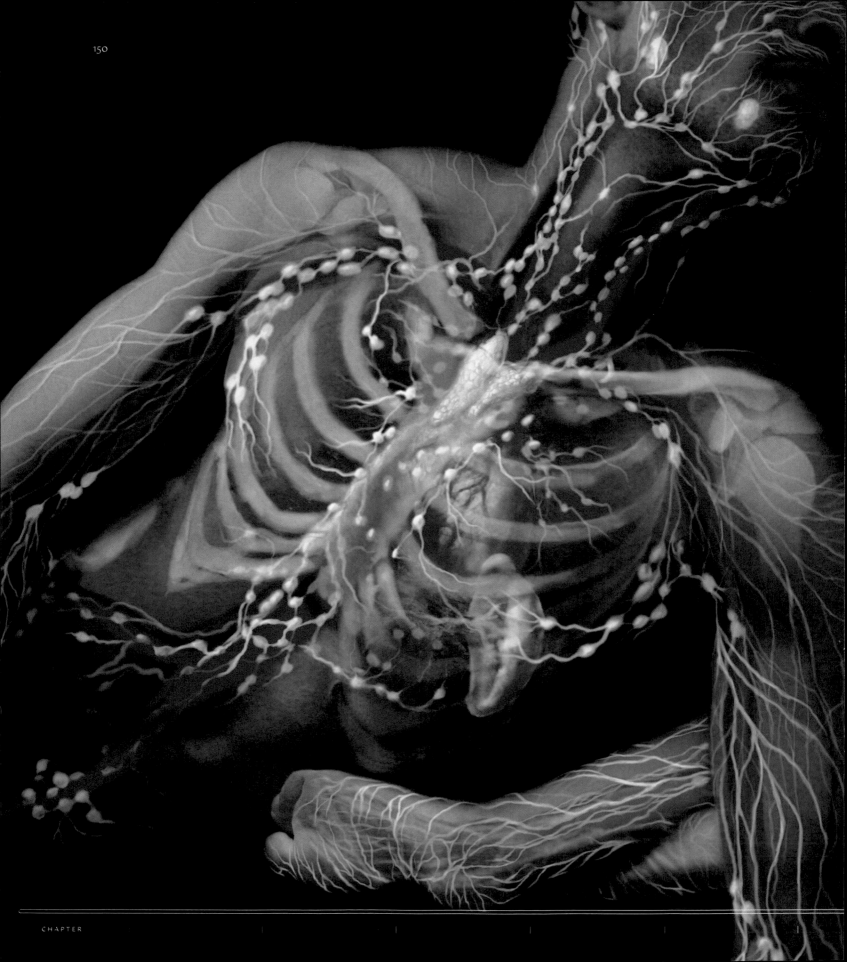

Designers of computer protection software (read: security geeks) exalt the immune system. It's their image of fulfillment, the focus of their longing. Foreign code in the form of a *virus* or *worm*; unanticipated code in the form of a *Trojan Horse* (a name also used for microbial hijackers like HIV); faulty bits of code—*bugs*; unauthorized users; corrupted data—like virtual pathogens, digital enemies threaten constantly from within and without. Programmers design counter-code to block and destroy them. Computer security systems are called "architectures for self-healing" and are increasingly modeled according to the concepts and principles behind our own inherent capacity to block disease.

The problem solved by the human immune system is the problem of determining "self" from "nonself." This "immunological conscience," as Sir Peter Medawar calls it, involves sophisticated notions of identity and protection—at cellular and molecular levels. Critical functions include being able to form a stable definition of what *self* is; prevent or detect, then eliminate, dangerous foreign activity (infection); recall previous infection; recognize new infection; and protect the immune system itself from attack.

Like baubles studding a pale brocade spanning the body—none larger than a fist, most smaller than a grape—the organs and glands of the immune and lymphatic systems do all this and more. Microsoft can only dream.

security

(immunological system)

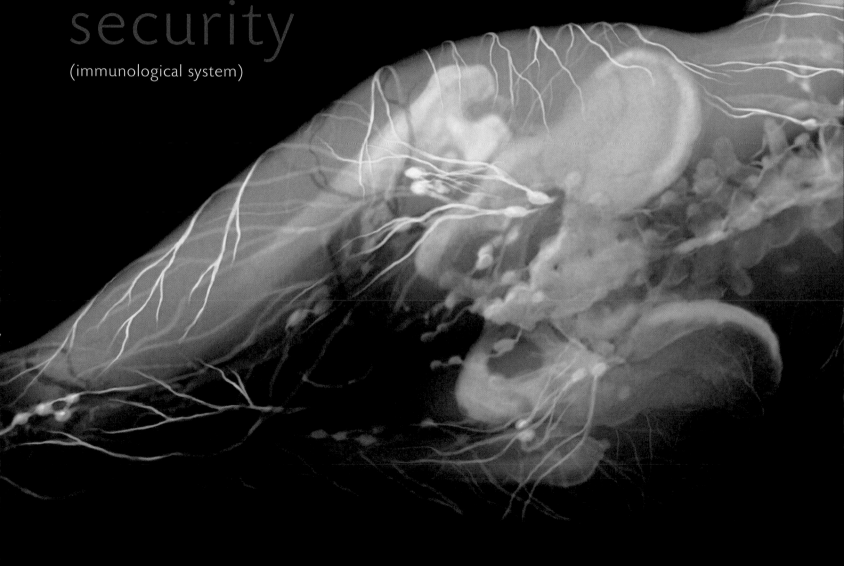

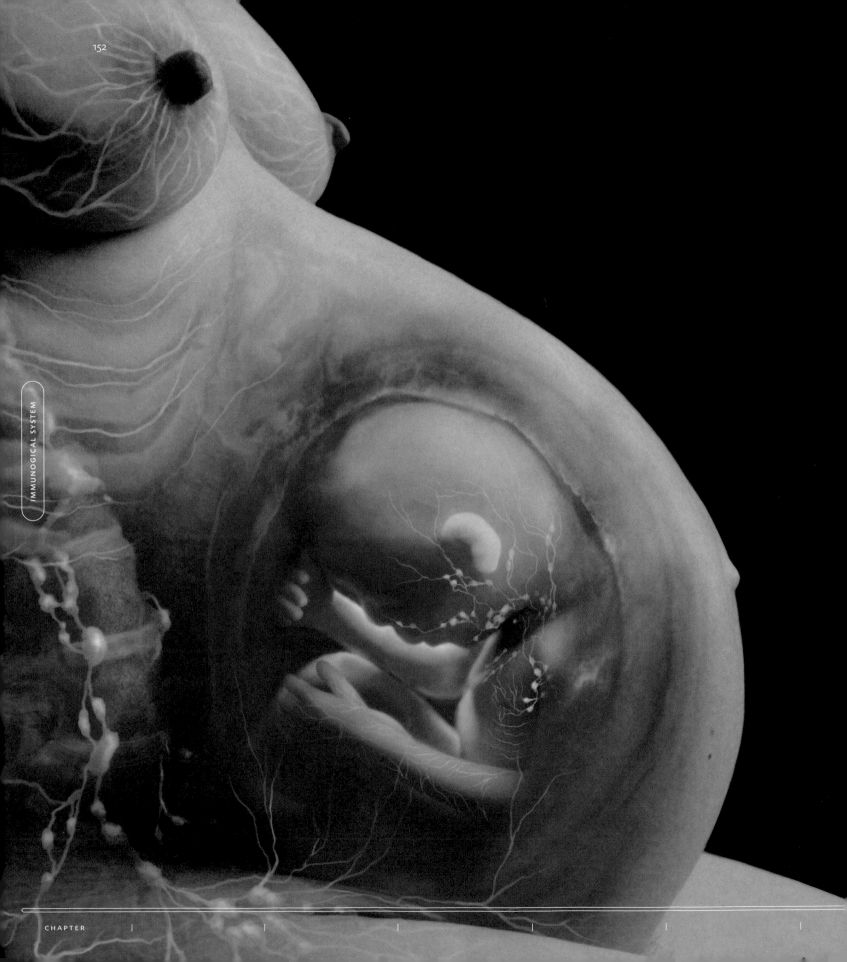

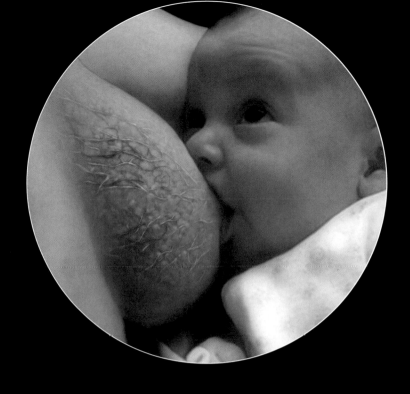

INITIAL DEFENSES

As a "security force" trained to identify and destroy chemical and biological attackers, the fetal immune system is fully mustered and positioned, but it remains to be programmed—that is, active immunity is developed, based on the body's ability to recognize threats against it. At birth, a mix of generically designed lymphocytes and immune proteins (antibodies) "downloaded" from the mother's blood temporarily enables newborns to resist harmful agents they haven't encountered before.

Ultimately, though, recognition is key.

Like alien computer code, antigens (protein markers on the surface of cells) distinguish pathogens, cancer cells, and other disease agents as "nonself." While nonspecific defenses provide protection against all pathogens, the immune system marshals attacks against specific pathogens and remembers them, filing their antigen structures in a kind of database so that if they attack again, the body can immediately respond by making antibodies. Though the system is exquisitely sensitive to differences, mistakes are sometimes made. Autoimmune diseases, often compared with friendly fire, result when our own cell antigens are wrongly identified as "nonself" and the system erroneously attacks them.

WHEN AN AIRBORNE
MICROBE
ENTERS THE NOSE

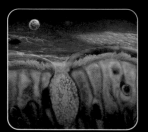

GOBLET CELLS OF THE
NASAL EPITHELIUM
SECRETE MUCOUS

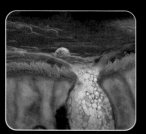

MICROBE IS TRAPPED
IN MUCOUS

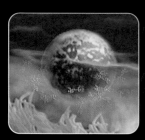

IMMUNE CELLS MIGRATE
TO MICROBE AND ATTACK
BY UNLEASING ENZYMES

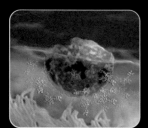

ENZYMES DEGRADE
MICROBE AND CILIA
SWEEP REMAINS AWAY

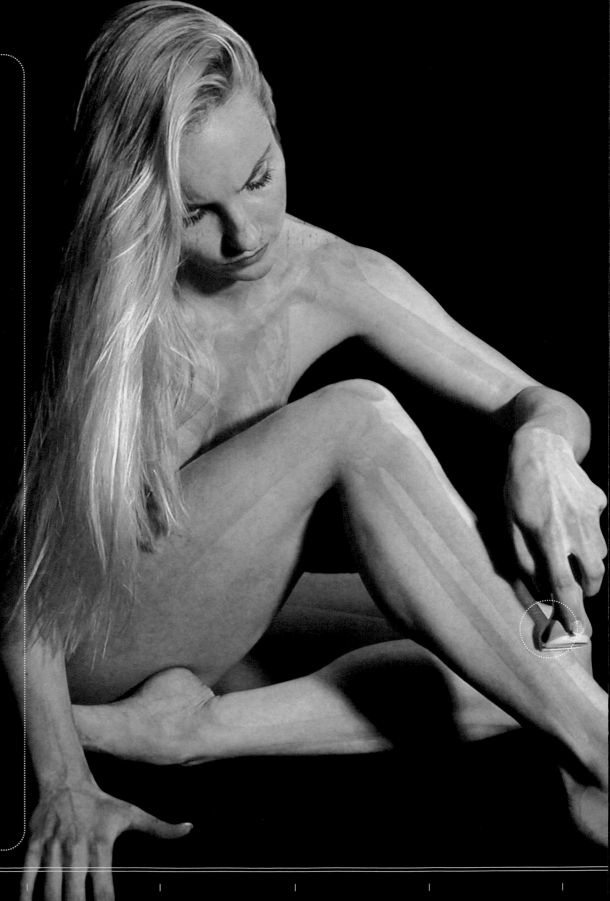

A reinforced shield girds the body perimeter: an outer barrier made of external membranes (intact skin and mucosa) that prevent the entry of microorganisms, backed up by a rapid-response capacity—inflammation. Imagine a computer, online, protected by a firewall and other security devices from the intrusion of countless new viruses and worms, with a back-up system in which Pac-Man-like bits of code burst out of nowhere to storm, block, and destroy anything that gets through.

Nicked while shaving, the skin is breached. Circulating in the underlying blood vessels are white blood cells that migrate to the site of the injury and release chemical signals that trigger inflammation, which occurs as bacteria-eating cells (neutrophils) arrive to inhibit opportunistic invaders. Chemical signals also call out short-lived white blood cells—monocytes—that mature on site into long-lived, hydralike macrophages, which have the ability to recognize and ingest all foreign antigens, and do the mopping up.

FRONT LINES

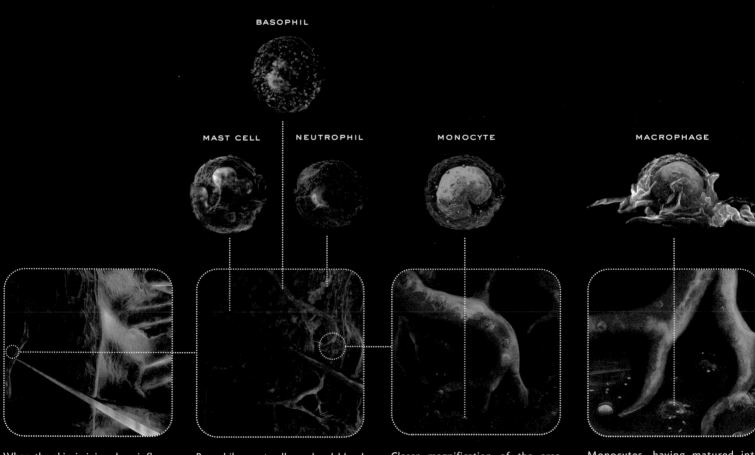

BASOPHIL

MAST CELL   NEUTROPHIL   MONOCYTE   MACROPHAGE

When the skin is injured an inflammatory response is triggered to rid the body of harmful invaders. To begin this response mast cells and basophils secrete chemical signals that promote blood flow to the area.

Basophils, mast cells, and red blood cells are joined within one hour of the injury by bacteria-eating cells called phagocytes, which include neutrophils and monocytes.

Closer magnification of the area shows phagocytes beginning to ingest pathogens and cellular debris.

Monocytes, having matured into macrophages (meaning "big-eaters"), continue to destroy pathogens and cellular debris by ingesting them, while the inflammation process begins to subside.

IMMUNOGICAL SYSTEM

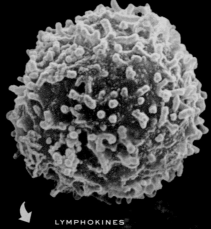

HELPER T CELL

FROM THYMUS

LYMPHOKINES

INITIAL CONTACT
USUALLY TAKES PLACE IN
LYMPH NODE OR SPLEEN.

LYMPHOKINES
STIMULATE INACTIVATED
MACROPHAGES.

UPON ACTIVATION, THE
MACROPHAGE REACHES
OUT TO BRING IN
BACTERIA AND DESTROY IT
THROUGH A PROCESS
CALLED PHAGOCYTOSIS.

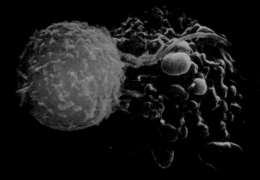

HUNDREDS OF MEMORY
T CELLS ARE ALSO
PRODUCED AND CIRCULATE
IN THE BLOODSTREAM
IN CASE OF A SIMILAR
FUTURE ATTACK.

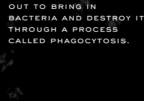
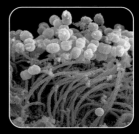
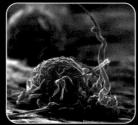

MACROPHAGE

BACTERIA

BATTLE PLAN "B"

If infection persists or spreads, specific immune responses are activated. Two types of armed forces (lymphocytes) work by recognizing the invader, launching a successful counter-strike, and remembering the invader's antigen structure (its digital signature, so to speak) in case of future infection.

Humoral immunity (RIGHT PAGE)—the part of the system that deploys antibodies directly against invaders, particularly bacteria and some viruses, such as attacking flu germs—involves a "lock and key" mechanism. The "arms" of Y-shaped antibodies, or immunoglobulins, possess unique, variable regions that bind to specific antigens carried by pathogens. Disabled by swarming antibodies, the pathogens are marked for destruction, then filtered out in the spleen.

Cellular immunity (LEFT PAGE) occurs when the body attacks cells infected by viruses or cancer cells by "reading" foreign antigen structures, then churning out killer cells that search out and lock onto identical forms in the body, destroying them with toxins.

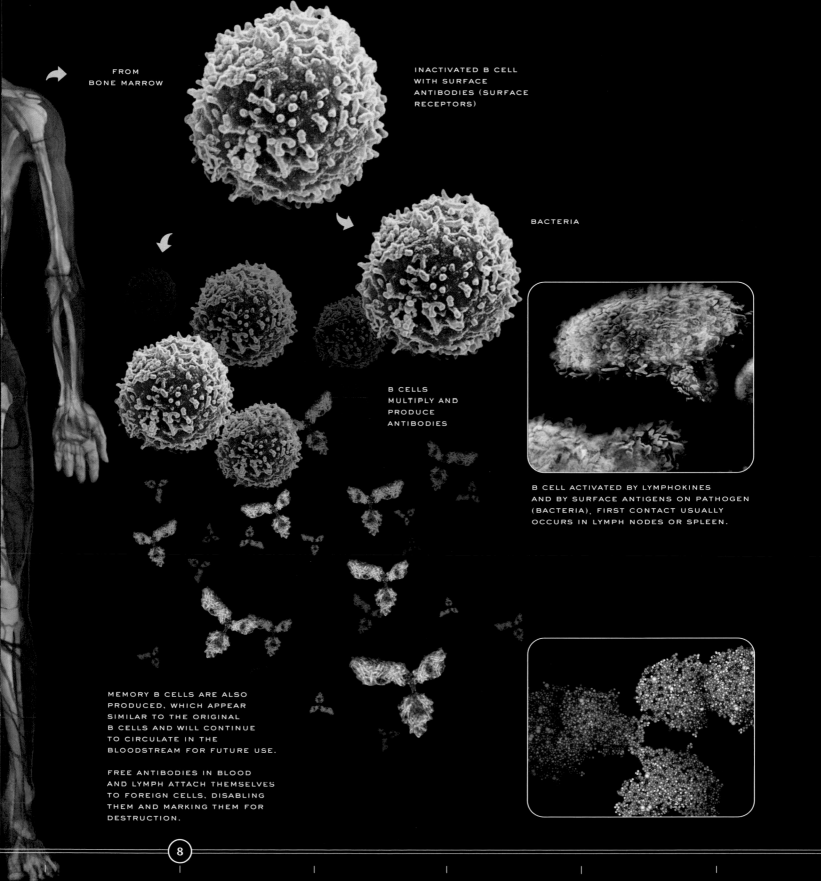

FROM
BONE MARROW

INACTIVATED B CELL
WITH SURFACE
ANTIBODIES (SURFACE
RECEPTORS)

BACTERIA

B CELLS
MULTIPLY AND
PRODUCE
ANTIBODIES

B CELL ACTIVATED BY LYMPHOKINES
AND BY SURFACE ANTIGENS ON PATHOGEN
(BACTERIA). FIRST CONTACT USUALLY
OCCURS IN LYMPH NODES OR SPLEEN.

MEMORY B CELLS ARE ALSO
PRODUCED, WHICH APPEAR
SIMILAR TO THE ORIGINAL
B CELLS AND WILL CONTINUE
TO CIRCULATE IN THE
BLOODSTREAM FOR FUTURE USE.

FREE ANTIBODIES IN BLOOD
AND LYMPH ATTACH THEMSELVES
TO FOREIGN CELLS, DISABLING
THEM AND MARKING THEM FOR
DESTRUCTION.

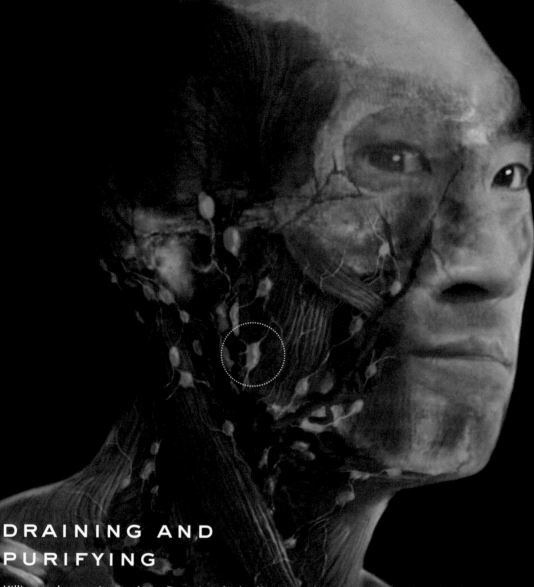

DRAINING AND PURIFYING

Killing pathogens is one thing. Dumping the bodies is another.

Lymph, which begins as fluid flowing between cells, is collected in special multivalve vessels that draw it away from the blood and toward centralized transfer stations called nodes (CROSS SECTION, RIGHT). Commonly referred to as "glands" by school nurses and others who explore children's necks and armpits for lumps, lymph nodes are masses of tissue that contain sinuses where white blood cells digest bacteria and debris, which is why they swell when we fight infection.

Tissue that supports lymphocyte activity is called lymphoid tissue. Packed in the spleen, the largest and most aggressive lymphoid organ, are long, barrel-like vascular channels lined by a nonporous layer of smooth cells, in turn supported by a noncellular "basement membrane" made up mostly of collagen. This structure permits easy passage of blood cell elements, which are filtered by macrophages that engulf bacteria, viruses, and worn-out red blood cells, then flushed out through the splenic vein.

Glands in the face and neck produce protective enzymes that patrol the tears, nasal passages, and mouth, destroying pathogens that come in contact with the eyes, or that we inhale or ingest. These drain into the spleen via the thoracic duct.

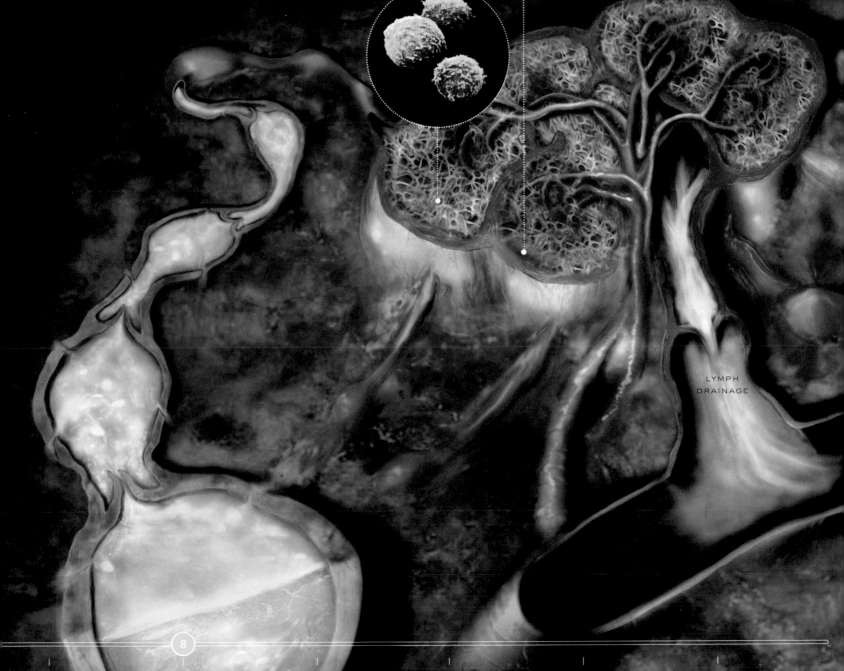

MACROPHAGE

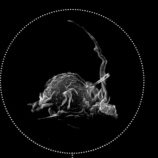

T-LYMPHOCYTES

LYMPH
DRAINAGE

8

MIRRORED IN NATURE

Basic units of the immune and lymphatic systems illustrate the 4 major stages of *pathogenocide*: 1) secretion of lethal materi- als (spongy, tubular salivary gland duct); 2) surface targeting of invaders (granular white blood cell); 3) engulfment (tentacled,

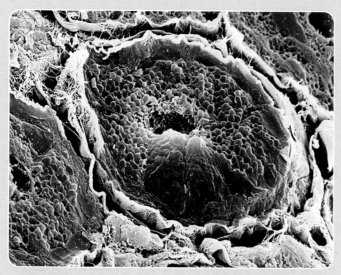

SALIVARY GLAND DUCT

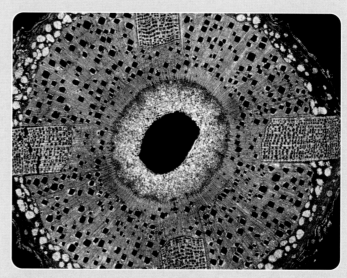

PLANT STEM

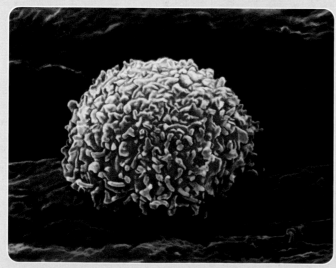

WHITE BLOOD CELL

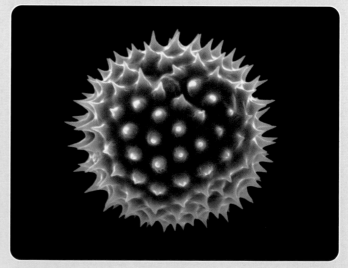

POLLEN CELL

Pac-Man-like, wandering macrophage); and 4) filtration and removal (string-latticelike lymph node tissue). Their architec- tures resemble others in nature where, though functions differ, similar motifs are applicable.

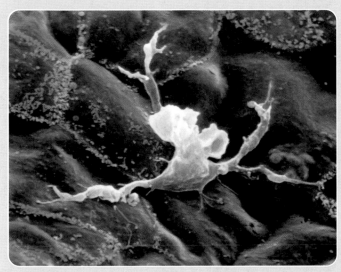

WANDERING MACROPHAGE

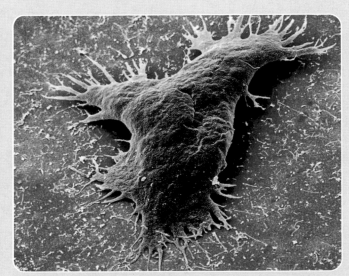

PROTOZOAN

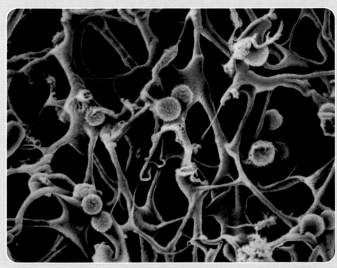

LYMPH NODE

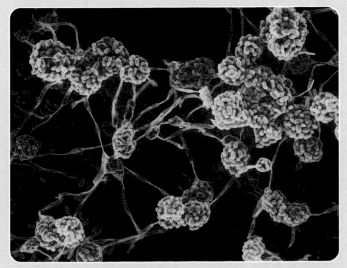

MOLD

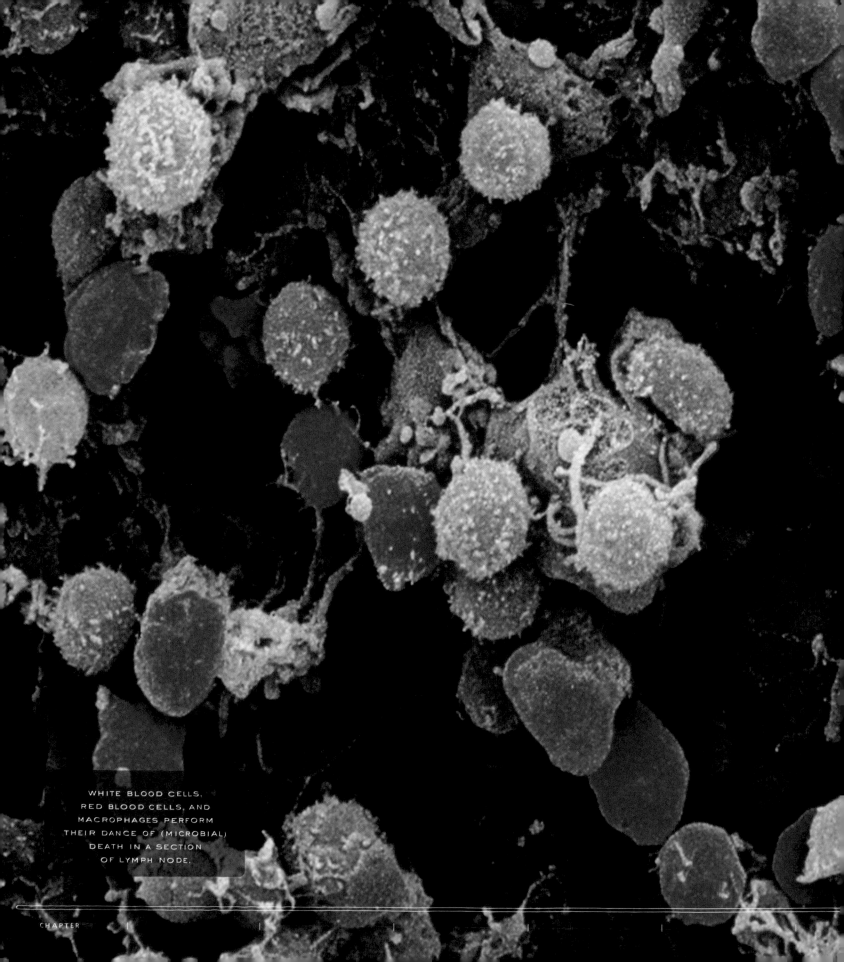

WHITE BLOOD CELLS,
RED BLOOD CELLS, AND
MACROPHAGES PERFORM
THEIR DANCE OF (MICROBIAL)
DEATH IN A SECTION
OF LYMPH NODE.

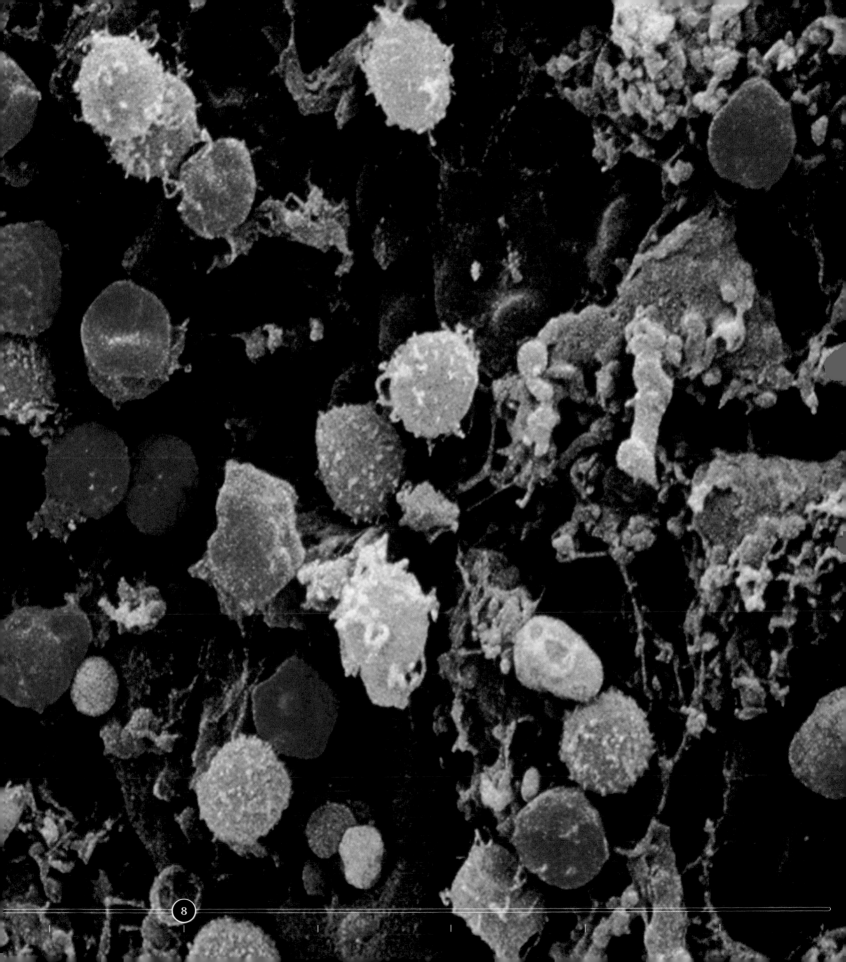

gas exchange

(respiratory system)

SLOW BURN

We breathe, therefore we are.

Not just at birth, when tiny and at times sodden lungs are ignited by their first scorching gulp of air and cry out. Nor only at the end, when we exhale for the last time and expire. Nor because, evolutionarily, the first eel-like creatures that dragged themselves onto land aeons ago are our ancestors.

Each of the body's trillions of cells needs oxygen to function and produce exhaust. While the body itself isn't a blimp, and has no capacity for storing gasses, it must draw them in and release them . . . continuously . . . rhythmically. The relentless exchange of gas molecules within cells in the production of physical energy—in essence, combustion—requires an involuntary apparatus of powerful intakes, vents, pumps, and gauges, attached to the bloodstream through the heart.

"'Tis her breathing that/Perfumes the chamber thus," Shakespeare wrote. That respiration, a gasworks, may also sweeten human encounters is one of life's more pleasurable enhancements, like a tender voice, sensual gaze, or tasty skin.

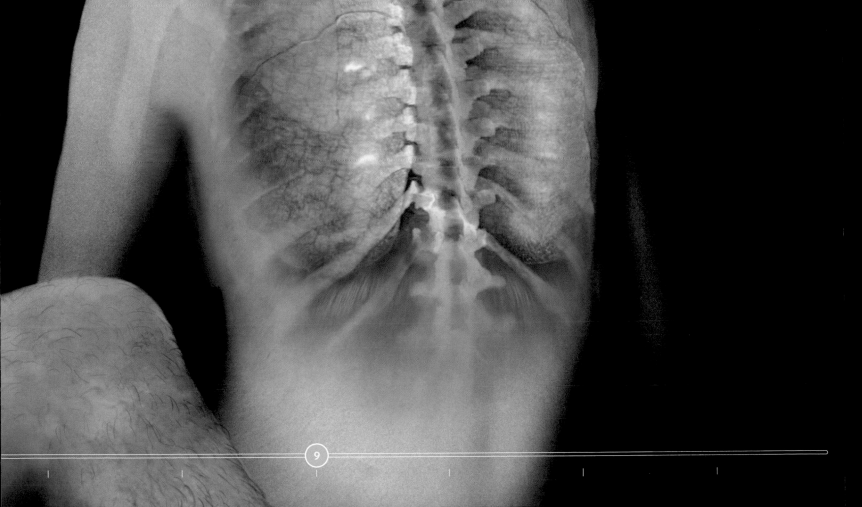

9

During pregnancy, oxygen arrives via the placenta; fetal lungs are dormant, albeit from early on they expand and contract, and contain amniotic fluid. Once the umbilical cord is cut at birth, carbon dioxide quickly builds up in the bloodstream, which signals the brain to activate the muscles of the diaphragm and rib cage to pull downward, which in turn allows the lungs room to fill like balloons. Taking in air for the first time, newborns cry out.

PUMP ACTIVATION

RESPIRATORY SYSTEM

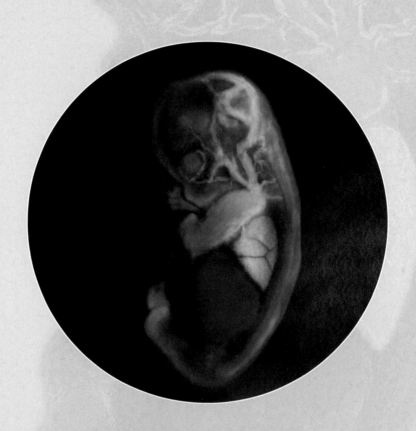

By adulthood, the rapid, unconscious exchange of gasses is voluminous—at rest, about 10 liters of air per minute, with the lungs filling and emptying every 4 to 5 seconds. Each breath is absorbed through a hollow treelike structure about the size of small bonsai. At the furthest reaches, oxygen molecules are removed via microscopic membranes that, if laid out flat, would equal a tennis court in size. Then, alternately, without missing a beat, the apparatus reverses direction, collecting and expelling an equal volume of carbon dioxide.

9

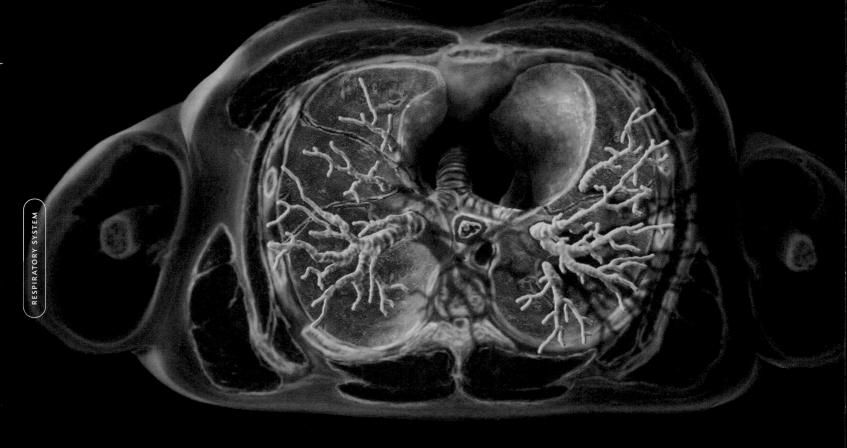

FULL SYSTEM

Muscular and compact, the respiratory system consists of branching tubes that perform 2 functions—one concerned with getting enormous volumes of air in and out of the body; and the other concentrated on getting oxygen into, carbon dioxide and water out of, the blood. How it does this in the space of 1 to 2 square feet of body cavity is a marvel of engineering and efficiency.

The core of the structure is the bronchial tree, an inverted system of airways in which the "trunk" is the wind-pipe and the "branches" are the subdividing passages that permeate the lungs. These branches split and split again until they are so numerous and so thin at their membranous tips that gas molecules cross into the blood through a network of capillaries which, laid end to end, would measure more than 1,000 miles. The accumulated physical force required to compress so much filtration into such a tight space is prodigious, as demonstrated by the highest recorded "sneeze speed"— about 100 miles per hour.

MAN

WOMAN

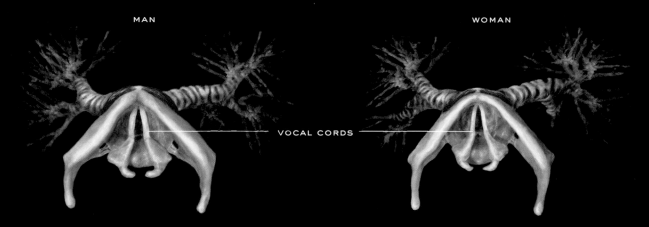

VOCAL CORDS

GENDER DIFFERENCES

Because men on average are larger than women, their vocal cords, as seen here from above, are thicker and their vocal tract longer, thus producing both lower tones and resonances: men tend to have deeper voices. But what about the significant size overlap between women and men? Why are the voices of large women higher than those of similarly sized men?

Part of the reason appears to be chemical—male vocal cords have more receptors for male sexual hormones. According to linguist James Fidelholtz, however, the prevail-ing reason may be social—men jut out their jaws, intention-ally dropping their voice registers, while women often speak "smilingly," stretching their lips to shorten their vocal tracts.

The Adam's apple is a bulge of the thyroid cartilage protruding under the skin. Its main purpose is to shield the larnyx. A secondary sexual trait like body hair, its growth is spurred by testosterone flowing through men's, and to a lesser extent, women's bodies.

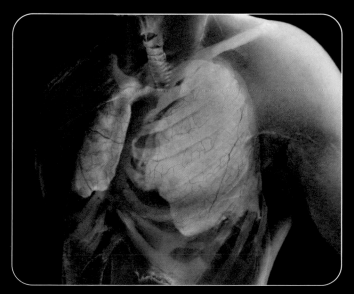

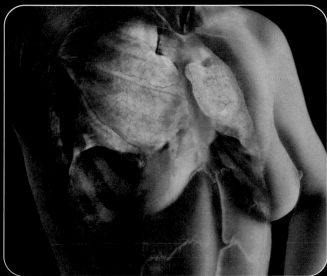

The amount of air that can be moved in and out of a person's lungs—so called vital capacity (VC)—is affected by age, height, and gender. Younger and taller people have larger VCs, while men exhibit more VC than women because their lungs are bigger, thus helping to explain why men grunt and bellow and find it easier to be blowhards.

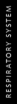

UPPER TRACT

Sarah Bernhardt described the voice as an instrument that a performer must learn to use "as if it were a limb." The "instrument," in fact, is the voice box (larynx), literally a musical organ in the neck. The size and shape of a plum, this framework of muscles, bone, and cartilage plays a crucial role in both speech and breathing.

Air entering the body is first warmed, cleaned, and humidified in the nasal area, then rapidly sucked into the voice box, the point at which the food and air shafts at the back of the mouth diverge. Because of its location, the voice box has 3 vital functions: control of the airflow during breathing, protection of the airway, and production of sound for speech.

Also because of its location—exposed and vulnerable, at the front of the neck—its inner works are heavily protected; muscles and tendons suspended from a U-shaped bone at the top of the larynx support it from above, elevating it during swallowing and speech; the tongue-shaped epiglottis keeps out food and liquids; a shield-shaped chunk of cartilage (Adam's apple) girds the anterior while the spine guards the rear; corrugated bands of cartilage hold its shape and prevent it from collapsing. It's within this chamber that loose pleats of tissue—the term "vocal cords" is somewhat misleading—extend from the interior wall into the airway, vibrating in the updraft when we exhale to create voice sounds.

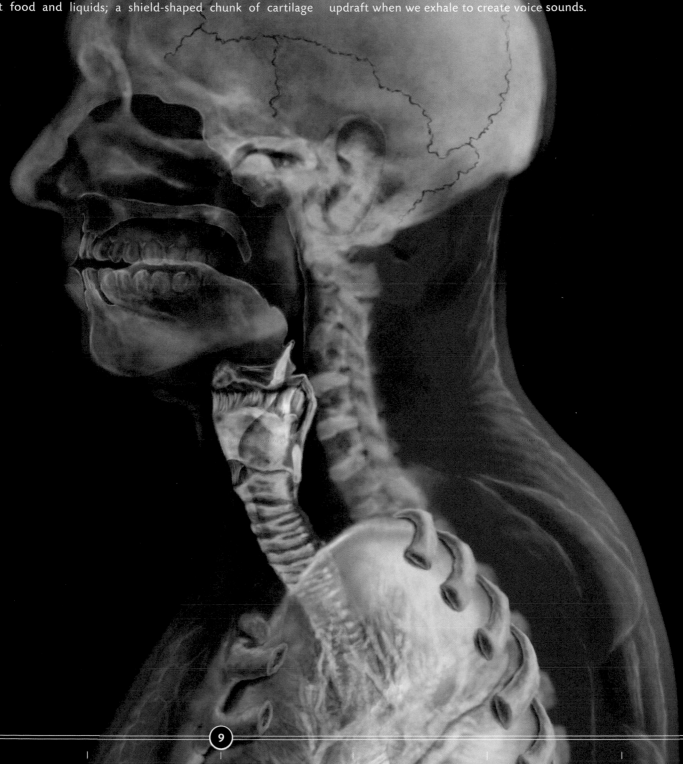

MECHANICS

The author Tom Wolfe often depicts male power in terms of chest muscles—massive "ripped" belts of rugged elastic, strapped across the upper torso like bandoliers. Lying beneath these powerful heaving muscles are the less pronounced muscles of respiration. The muscles located between the ribs and below the lungs do the job of pulling the lungs outwards and downwards. As the lungs expand, the pressure inside them is reduced, and they suck in air. During extreme inhalation, the neck muscles also contract. Picture an exhausted marathoner at the finish line—head back, throat open, intercostal muscles (those between the ribs) engorged and rippling.

Less in evidence—behind the scenes, so to speak—is the diaphragm, the sheet of muscle tucked between the thorax and abdomen. When we breathe in, the diaphragm contracts and pushes downwards; when we breathe out, it relaxes and is pushed up into a dome shape by the lower digestive organs, compressing the lungs. As pressure rises in the (now smaller) chest cavity, we exhale, equalizing the air pressure with the outside and restarting the cycle.

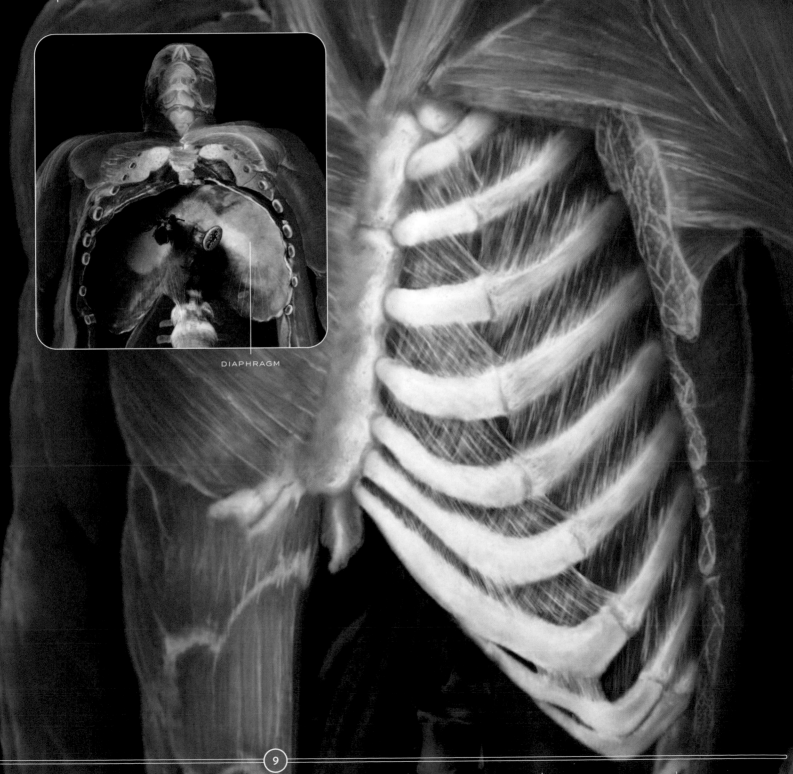

DIAPHRAGM

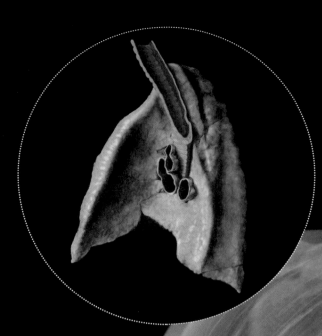

INSIDE VIEW OF RIGHT LUNG

The substance of the lung is dilatable and extensible like the tinder made from a fungus. But it is spongy, and if you press it, it yields to the force which compresses it, and if the force is removed, it increases again to its original size. —Leonardo da Vinci

OUTSIDE VIEW OF RIGHT LUNG

THE LUNGS

Dissecting cadavers night after night in the fifteenth century, da Vinci discerned the accordionlike mechanical process of breathing but not the actual mechanism at work in creating a breath. That mechanism—rapid gas exchange and cellular respiration—wasn't understood for another 300 years. Only then did the structural design of the lungs, and its vital connections to the central nervous system and heart (TOP INSETS), become clear.

Only about 10 percent of the lung is occupied by solid tissue. The rest is filled with air and blood. Lung tissue must therefore be sheer enough to allow gas to pass through it yet

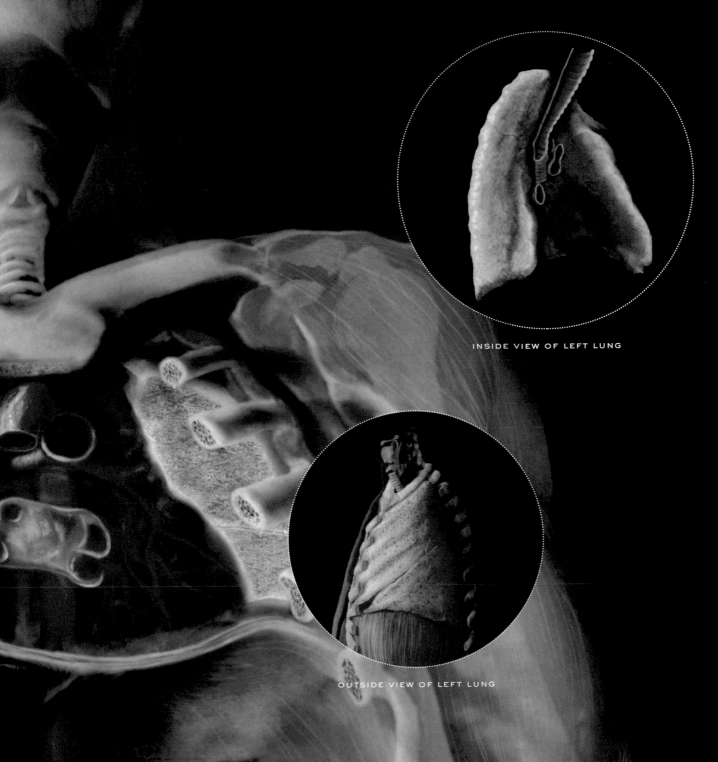

INSIDE VIEW OF LEFT LUNG

OUTSIDE VIEW OF LEFT LUNG

strong enough to keep the separate balloonlike portions—lobes—from collapsing (BOTTOM INSETS). Its asymmetrical shape—the right lung consists of 3 lobes, the left of 2—allows room for the heart, which each minute pumps the entire blood volume of the body (about 5 liters) through the lungs.

Gas exchange takes 0.25 seconds, or a third of the total transit time of a red blood cell through the area.

Surrounding the lungs, and enabling them to expand and shrink smoothly with each breath, are two elastic sacs separated by a layer of lubricating fluid.

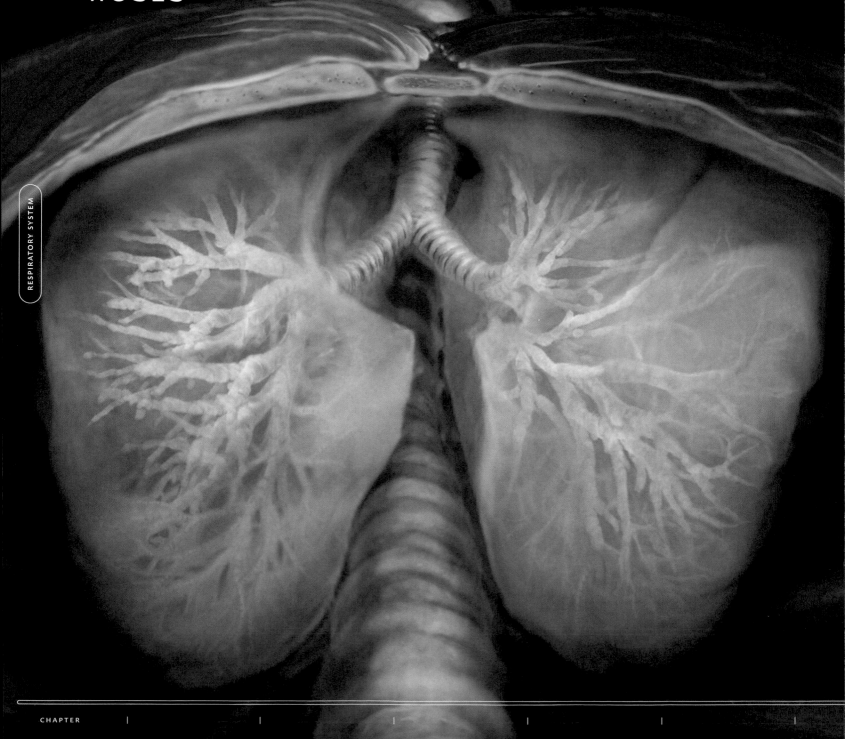

In 1953, an American company called Plastiflex introduced the first crush-proof hose. Vinyl tubing ribbed with wire, the hose was pliable enough to bend at sharp angles yet sturdy enough not to be squashed. It became the industry standard for products ranging from vacuum cleaners to washing machines and swimming pools, and it borrows its design from the human windpipe and its main tributaries.

C-shaped bands of cartilage jacket the major airways,

TOUGH, FLEXIBLE
HOSES

preventing them from collapsing under pressure and thereby guaranteeing air supply. Not merely the durable fiber of the bronchial tree's "bark"—its tough outer coating—the rings also serve as a type of exoskeleton, a scaffolding embedded in the airways' walls for support. As the trunk splits into 2 main bronchi (Greek for "windpipe"), 1 for each lung, then split again and again until there are about 30,000 twiglike bronchioles on each side, the ring pattern gradually disappears.

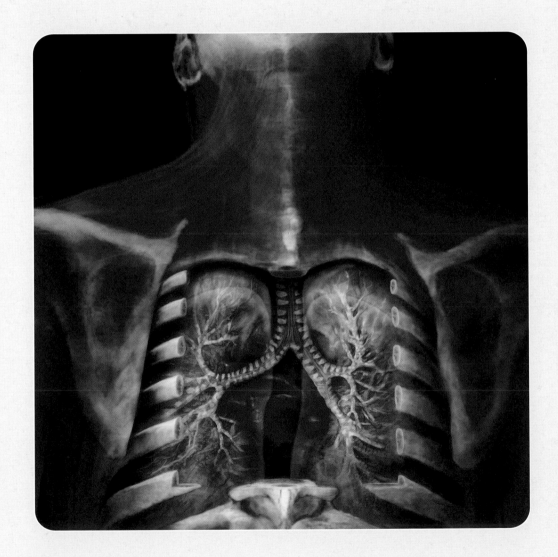

178

Clustered like grapes, the *alveoli* (Latin for "small hollows") are intertwined with microscopic vinelike blood vessels. As breathing increases the air pressure inside each sac, the natural tendency of molecules to move randomly from areas of high concentration to low ones quickly sends oxygen bursting into the blood while evacuating potentially poisonous carbon dioxide in the opposite direction. The balloon leaks from every pore yet never deflates.

Recently, University of Pittsburgh surgeon and immunologist Dr. Brack Hattler introduced an artificial breathing device that operates similarly. Called IMO (intravenous or implantable membrane oxygenator), Hattler's artificial lung consists of a balloon-tipped catheter connected to a vacuum pump. The balloon is packed with a thousand fibers of semipermeable membrane. Pulsating about 300 times a minute, it inflates and deflates while also stirring the blood, creating the conditions for high-speed diffusion. Noting the potential improvement over conventional mechanical respirators, which draw blood outside the body, run it through gas exchangers and heaters, then pump it back inside with cell-tearing force, *Wired* magazine dubbed Hattler "Puff Daddy."

GAS EXCHANGE

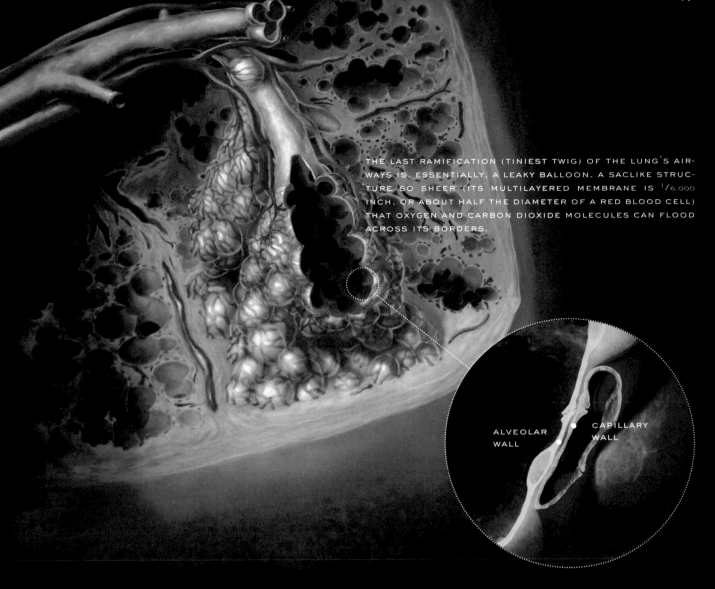

THE LAST RAMIFICATION (TINIEST TWIG) OF THE LUNG'S AIR-
WAYS IS, ESSENTIALLY, A LEAKY BALLOON, A SACLIKE STRUC-
TURE SO SHEER (ITS MULTILAYERED MEMBRANE IS $^1/_{6,000}$
INCH, OR ABOUT HALF THE DIAMETER OF A RED BLOOD CELL)
THAT OXYGEN AND CARBON DIOXIDE MOLECULES CAN FLOOD
ACROSS ITS BORDERS.

ALVEOLAR
WALL

CAPILLARY
WALL

PULMONARY VASCULATURE

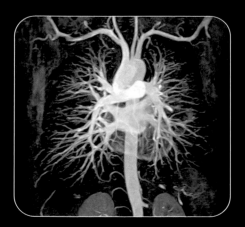

In a circulatory sense, the lungs are a mini-Bizarro version of what happens throughout the body. Blood moving away from the heart through the pulmonary arteries is dark, spent—deoxygenated—while blood returning to the heart through the pulmonary veins is bright red and oxygen-rich.

After spent blood enters the right atrium of the heart, it is squeezed into the right ventricle, then pumped into the lungs—at a resting rate of 5 liters per minute. From here, the main artery branches and branches again, ferrying cells throughout the lung tissue, including major areas above the rib cage. Like telephone lines along a rail bed, the arteries track the path of the bronchi and bronchioles, terminating in a capillary bed that permeates—and clings to—the alveoli. As the blood leaves the alveoli, other capillaries merge to form progressively larger veins, which empty into 2 major veins that return oxygenated blood to the heart.

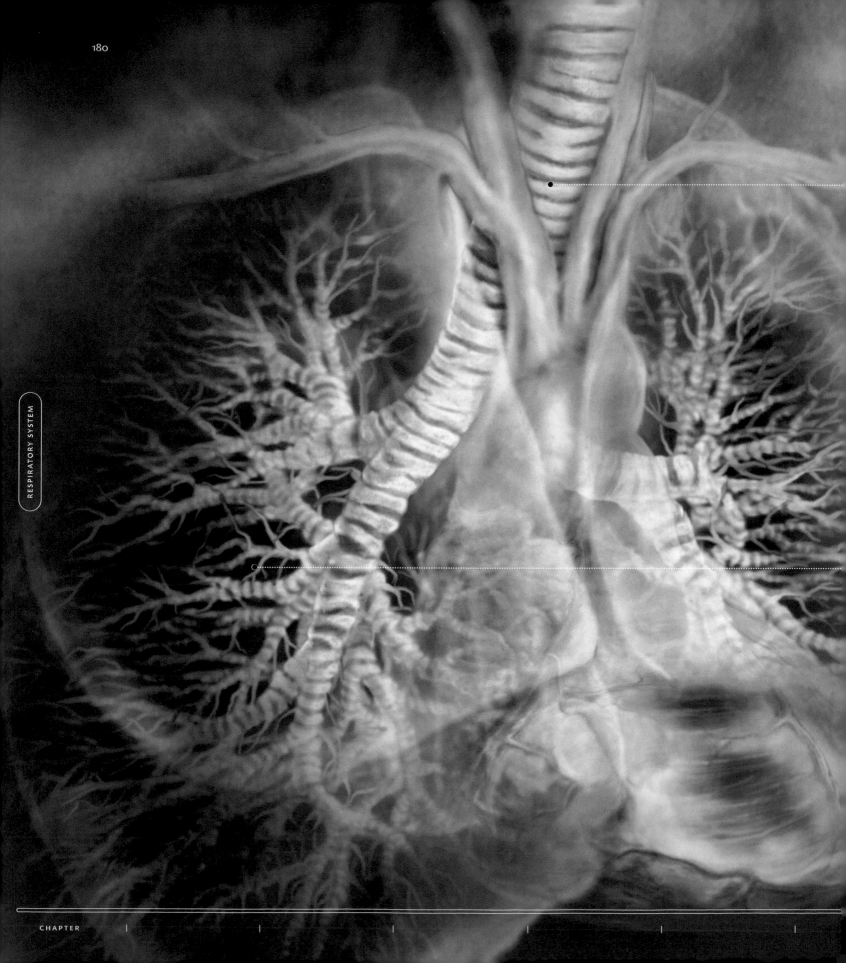

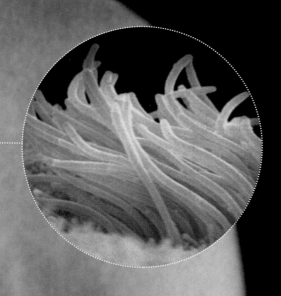

LIKE INFINITESIMAL MOPS, CILIA (LITTLE HAIRS) PROJECT FROM THE CELLS LINING THE TRACHEA. SWAYING RHYTHMICALLY, THEY WAFT DUST-LADEN MUCUS UP TO THE THROAT, WHERE IT CAN BE SWALLOWED OR SPAT OUT.

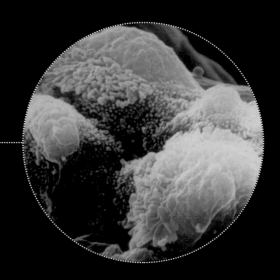

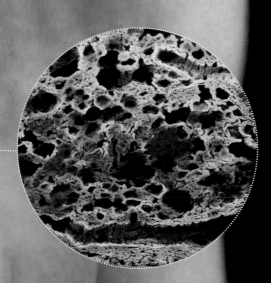

MICROSCOPIC ANATOMY

The smallest structures of the respiratory system share a common need—to optimize the speed and efficiency with which gas molecules move back and forth between them. Dense capillary beds, each a single cell thick, gird the bulb-shaped alveoli (MIDDLE AND BOTTOM CROSS SECTION), which are essentially bubbles packed in bubbles, a design that both speeds diffusion and provides physical support. Sustaining a continuous airflow to the alveoli is a hollow trunk and branch network, built much the same way as a sea anemone, broccoli floret, or oak.

MIRRORED IN NATURE

Long, cylindrical, divided into ringlike segments for structural stability, the trachea resembles nothing so much as an earthworm—a straight-line tube within a tube. Air sacs in the lungs are girded by wrinkled, crosslinked membranes, much like spores, which are encased in multilayered protein shells that lock their cargo of DNA into a stable state. The densely ramifying bronchial

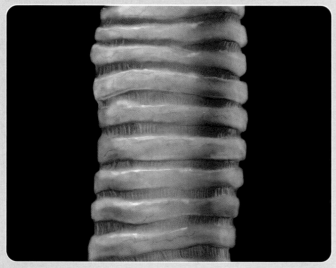

CARTILAGINOUS RINGS OF TRACHEA

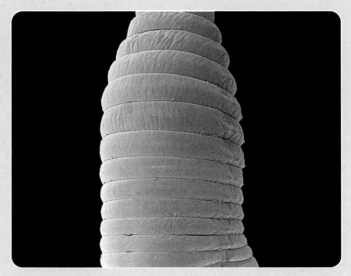

COMMON EARTHWORM

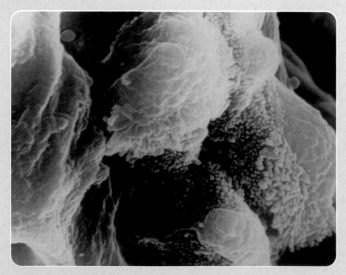

ALVEOLAR SACS IN LUNGS

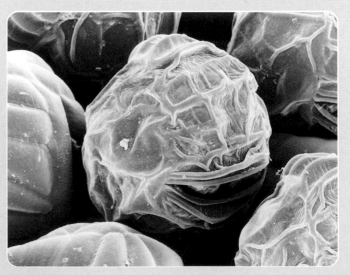

FERN SPORES

tree, which carries air to the alveoli, reflects the denuded branches of a tree in winter. Like lung tissue, leaves—the chief organs of photosynthesis—are honeycombed with air space, allowing access of CO_2 to individual cells.

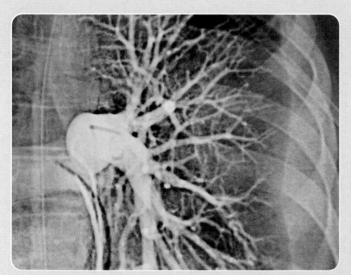

BRONCHIAL BRANCHES

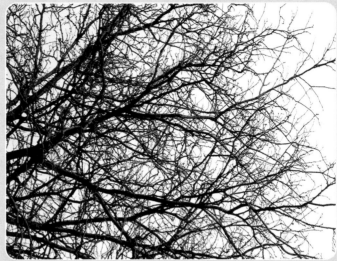

LEAFLESS TREE BRANCHES

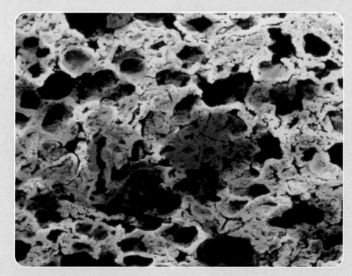

LUNG TISSUE AND AIRWAYS

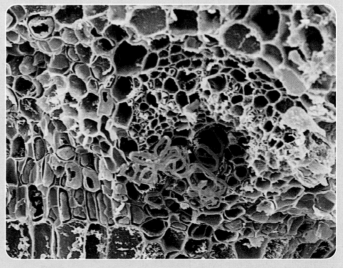

CROSS SECTION OF LEAF

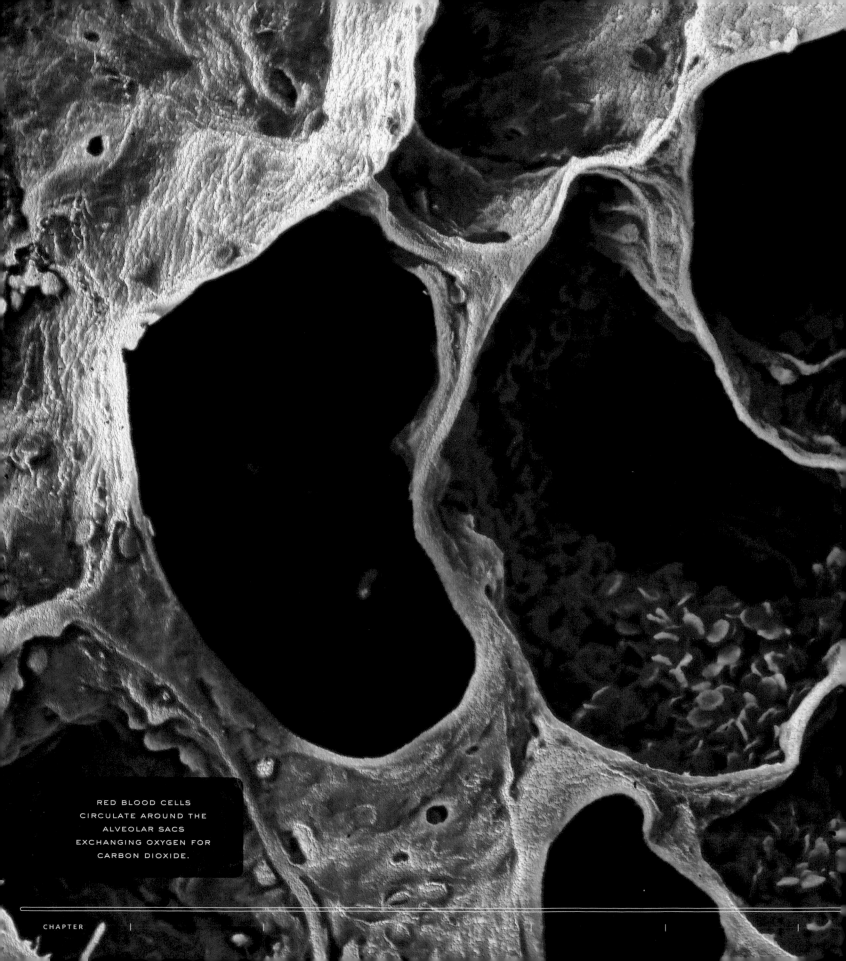

RED BLOOD CELLS
CIRCULATE AROUND THE
ALVEOLAR SACS
EXCHANGING OXYGEN FOR
CARBON DIOXIDE.

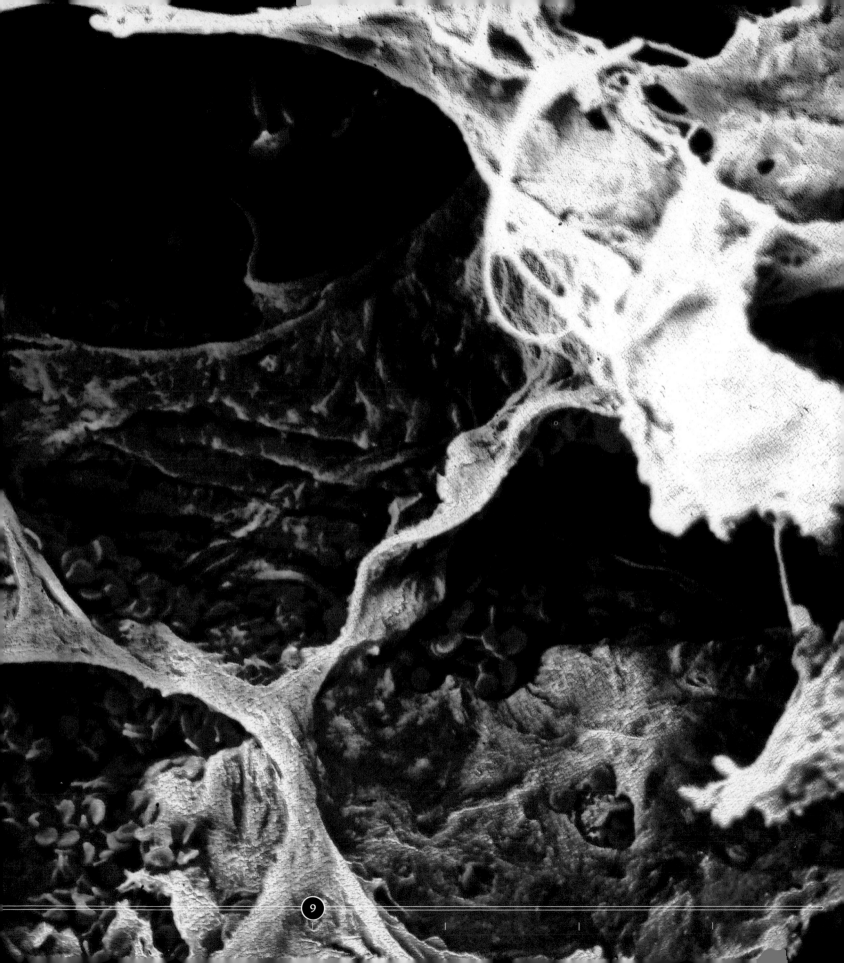

solid intake/
waste removal

(digestive system)

Snaking smoothly from lips to lower bowel, the digestive tract reverses the normal course of evolution, breaking down complex biological structures into simpler ones. In 2001, its twisting architecture of tubes, valves, and reservoirs inspired a Los Angeles–based mixed-media sculptor named Tim Hawkinson to build a giant self-playing reed organ. By inflating 12 organically shaped clear balloons, some 20 feet high, with pressurized air through a central ductwork of polyethylene tubing, Hawkinson created an instrument that looked—and could blast, toot, and growl—like a gargantuan digestive system. His Uberorgan, as he called it, was effectively the world's biggest bagpipe, a football field from end to end.

Our own gastrointestinal tract is 26 to 30 feet long, and though at times embarrassing, similarly expressive. The core is a long, looping tube with a lubricated lining—the alimentary canal—operated by muscle power. Festooned along its length are a varied group of task-oriented "accessory" organs, from teeth and tongue to gallbladder and pancreas. Think of a pulsing disassembly line where successive precision machines cut, crush, whisk, sort, convert, and discard waves of complex nutrients in a high-throughput process for extracting fuel molecules one at a time.

It's estimated that the average person eats more than 20 tons of food in a lifetime. Recent obesity studies show a higher prevalence in women, who because they are generally smaller and less muscular than men, burn calories at a slower rate, and whose eating behaviors and energy storage needs are understood as advantages in bearing and raising children.

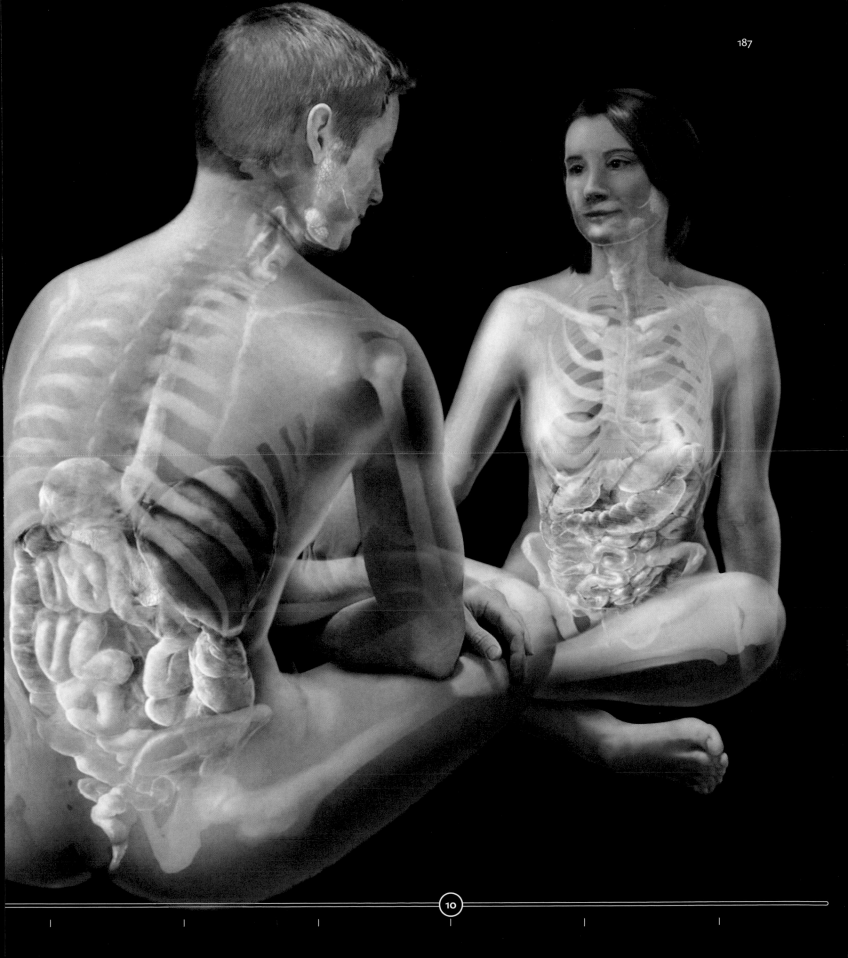

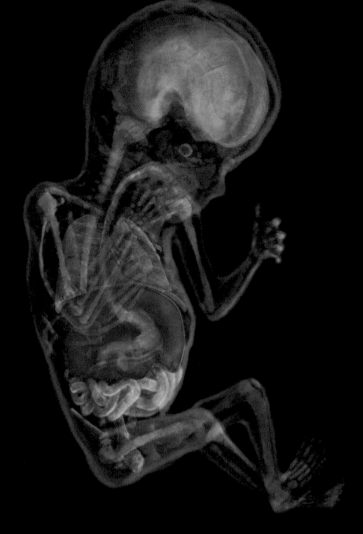

ASSEMBLY

The digestive system (unlike, say, the circulatory system) has no current job to do *in utero*. Except for the liver, which fills in temporarily as a blood factory until enough bone marrow is formed, its embryonic structures need only to form and be prepared, like armed forces in peacetime. In their primitive stage, the organs of the digestive tract make up one continuous tube that is attached to the abdominal walls by two membranous sheets. As the organs develop, they bud off from their respective locations and embark on a bustling journey of jostling, twisting, and coiling before migrating to their final positions. The surrounding membranes of some of these organs—the pancreas, duodenum, and ascending and descending stretches of the colon—fuse with the membranes at the rear wall of the body, permanently anchoring them into position. Thus mounted, the organs of the gastrointestinal tract can writhe independently of each other and absorb substantial pummeling, from inside and out.

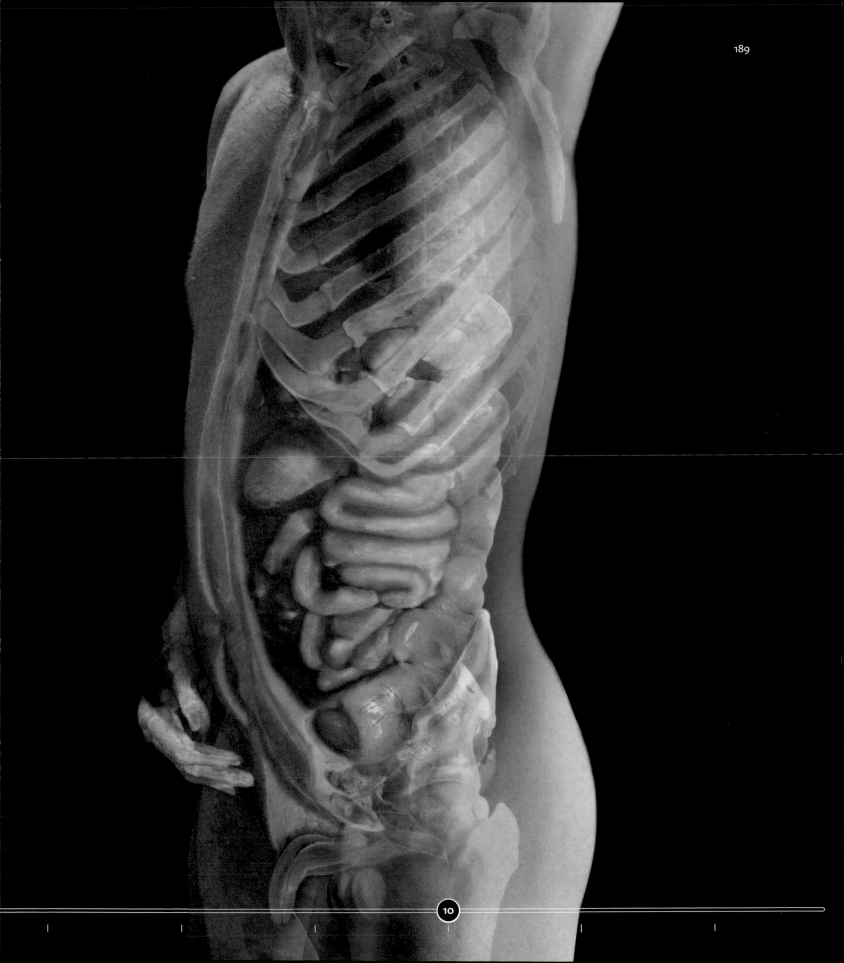

DIGESTIVE SYSTEM

FULL SYSTEM

Top to bottom, the digestive systems of men and women consist of all the same structures, in the same proportions. There are a few exceptions: the jaw and teeth of the male are somewhat larger, adapting perhaps to the role of provider; and the organs of the lower intestinal tract of the female settle a bit lower and wider due to the shape of the female pelvis. Yet with eating- and drinking-related chemical processes, sex matters often decisively. For instance, females appear to empty both solids and liquids more slowly than males; male livers secrete twice as much of certain chemicals that transport many toxic molecules, including drugs, out of cells; and females produce less of the gastric enzyme that breaks down alcohol in the stomach. After drinking the same amount, women have higher blood-alcohol content than men, even after allowing for size differences. Men and women differ as well in how their bodies metabolize drugs, resulting in different therapeutic responses and long-term side effects.

GENDER DIFFERENCES

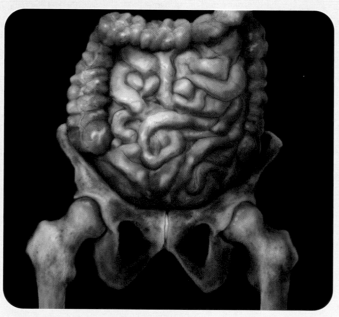

MAN

WOMAN

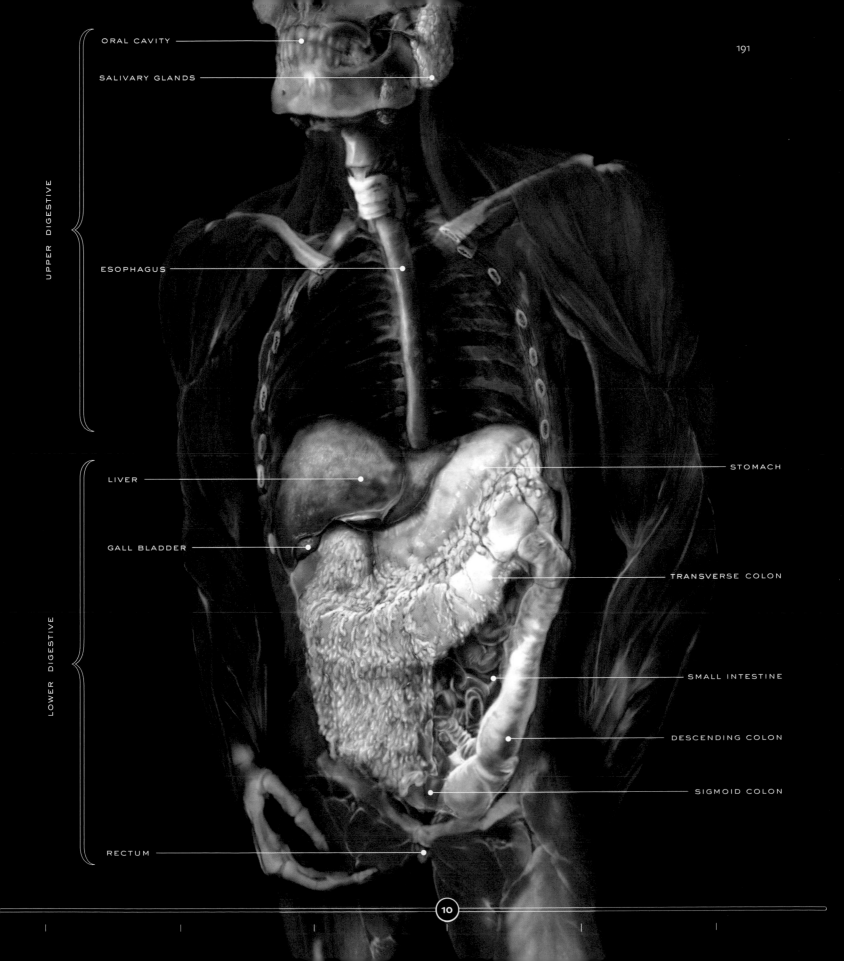

ORAL CAVITY

SALIVARY GLANDS

UPPER DIGESTIVE

ESOPHAGUS

STOMACH

LIVER

GALL BLADDER

TRANSVERSE COLON

LOWER DIGESTIVE

SMALL INTESTINE

DESCENDING COLON

SIGMOID COLON

RECTUM

ENTRYWAY

As a flexible, oval-shaped antechamber where the front doors flap open and shut and the sides rock up and down; where pounding rows of ivory spikes and anvils tear and crush whatever comes in; where water and corrosive chemicals gush from behind walls and under the floor; and where a spade of solid muscle tamps and rolls whatever comes by into a wet clump and dumps it down into darkness—the mouth is designed mechanically like an evil funhouse.

Every structure serves a different purpose, and solves a different problem. The lips—"roses on a stalk," Shakespeare called them—conceal a voluntary, sphincterlike muscle that acts not only to open and seal an orifice but also to protrude sensuously and explode into a grin, an asset on any face. Thirty-two permanent teeth—some chisel-shaped with sharp edges, some pointed, and some flat and slightly grooved—cut, tear, and grind up substances from beef jerky to grape nuts. On the surface of the tongue and at the back of the throat are thousands of microscopic eruptions that look like peeled oranges with little hairs sticking up—antennae for detecting flavor molecules. Sweet registers at the tip, salty in the middle, bitter at the back.

Three pairs of pepper-shaped glands, under the chin and in front of the ears, lubricate the process by washing it all down with what we call spit. The problem, from the funhouse

DIGESTIVE SYSTEM

RINGLIKE MUSCLES IN THE ESOPHAGUS CONTRACT RHYTHMICALLY TO PUSH THE FOOD DOWN TOWARD THE STOMACH, AN INVOLUNTARY MASSAGING MOTION SO POWERFUL THAT IT'S POSSIBLE TO SWALLOW FOOD EVEN WHILE HANGING UPSIDE DOWN.

EPIGLOTTIS

SALIVARY GLAND

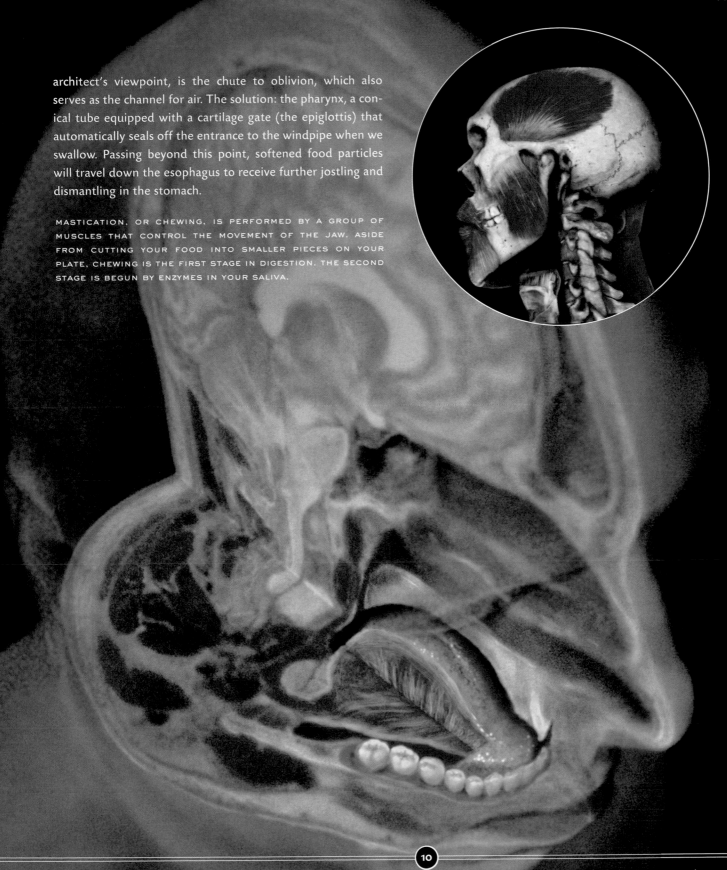

architect's viewpoint, is the chute to oblivion, which also serves as the channel for air. The solution: the pharynx, a conical tube equipped with a cartilage gate (the epiglottis) that automatically seals off the entrance to the windpipe when we swallow. Passing beyond this point, softened food particles will travel down the esophagus to receive further jostling and dismantling in the stomach.

MASTICATION, OR CHEWING, IS PERFORMED BY A GROUP OF MUSCLES THAT CONTROL THE MOVEMENT OF THE JAW. ASIDE FROM CUTTING YOUR FOOD INTO SMALLER PIECES ON YOUR PLATE, CHEWING IS THE FIRST STAGE IN DIGESTION. THE SECOND STAGE IS BEGUN BY ENZYMES IN YOUR SALIVA.

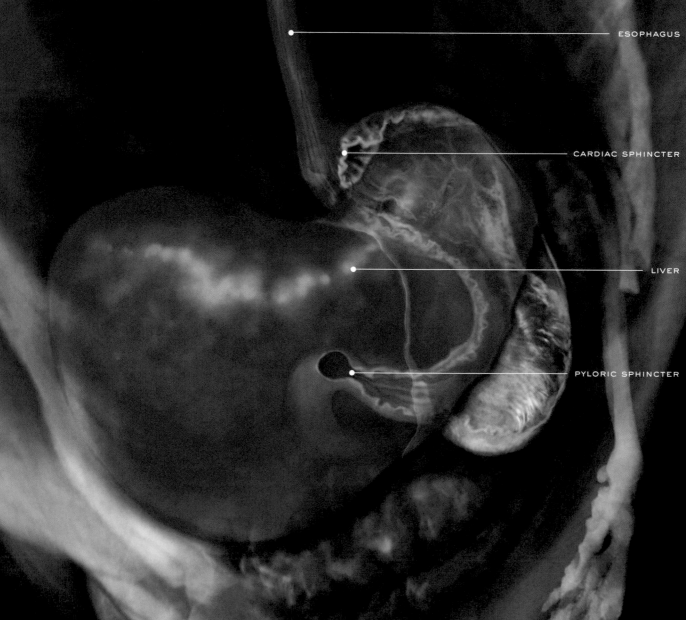

Early nineteenth-century European physicians, having no way to witness digestion at work, argued whether the stomach ground food up, cooked it, or reduced it chemically. "Some will have it that the stomach is a mill, others that it is a fermenting vat, others again that it is a stew pot," an English surgeon observed. Then, in 1822, a Canadian fur trapper survived a shotgun blast that ripped a $2\,^{1}/_{2}$-inch hole in his stomach that wouldn't close, and the U.S. Army surgeon who treated him, Dr. William Beaumont, conducted experiments through the open wound, dangling pieces of food into the cavity and observing their disintegration over time. Beaumont, known as the father of gastric physiology, showed that gastric juice has solvent properties and needs heat to digest. He also noted—the trapper got irritable at having his food removed during observation—that anger can impede digestion.

A MILL, A VAT,
A STEW POT

DIGESTIVE SYSTEM

ESOPHAGUS

CARDIAC SPHINCTER

LIVER

PYLORIC SPHINCTER

FOLDS OF THE STOMACH
INCREASE SURFACE
AREA FOR MORE
EFFICIENT DIGESTION.

The stomach, an inflatable J-shaped bag tucked under the ribs, is lined with a corrugated wall wrapped in 3 cross-hatched bands of muscle and encased in an elastic membrane. Glands in the dense folds along the interior surface produce about 6 pints of highly acidic gastric juice each day, which, along with the rolling motion of the muscle layers, make the stomach a kind of churn. Smaller than a fist when empty, it can inflate to 20 times its size after a meal, processing and storing up to several gallons daily of a thick, creamy mix of food and gastric juice called *chyme*. A sphincter at the bottom end regulates the release of the semidigested chyme into the intestines. The acid is strong enough to dissolve small pieces of bone, yet doesn't digest the stomach itself because the lining is covered with protective mucus.

LEFT LOBE OF LIVER

RIGHT LOBE OF LIVER

GALLBLADDER

CHEMICAL PLANT

Eighty percent of the cells in the liver are hepatocytes—microscopic chemical factories run by robotic machines. It is here that, among other things, blood sugar is regulated, fat and protein are metabolized, bile is produced, vitamins and minerals are stored, and blood is detoxified. A high degree of structural organization is key.

Distinctly round, hepatocytes are packed with organelles, storage particles, and especially enzymes. Nutrients and toxins arrive from the digestive tract, blood products from the spleen, and endocrine secretions from the pancreas, as well as oxygenated blood from the heart. The enzymes cut and reassemble the molecules, producing in turn vital proteins and digestive enzymes that need to be transported in 2 directions; 1 back to the bloodstream, the other to the intestines. Handling the flow—half the body's blood courses through the liver at any given time, and it produces about a quart of bile a day—requires optimal contact with 3 massive networks of sluices and drains. In other words, extreme plumbing.

Hence the liver's structure (LOWER RIGHT). The hepatocytes are organized into plates just 1 or 2 cell layers thick, separated by spaces filigreed with capillaries and "ductules." The plates are stacked, like records on a turntable, in honeycombed columns called lobules, which are bordered by intertwining branches delivering blood, hormones, and digestive secretions such as bile. Each lobule, as complicated structurally as a skyscraper, measures the length of a sesame seed, and nearly 1 million of them—a megalopolis—make up the liver, which is about the size and shape of a flattened football. The second largest organ in the body after the skin, the liver is able to regenerate after injuries, growing back even if two thirds of its cells have been destroyed.

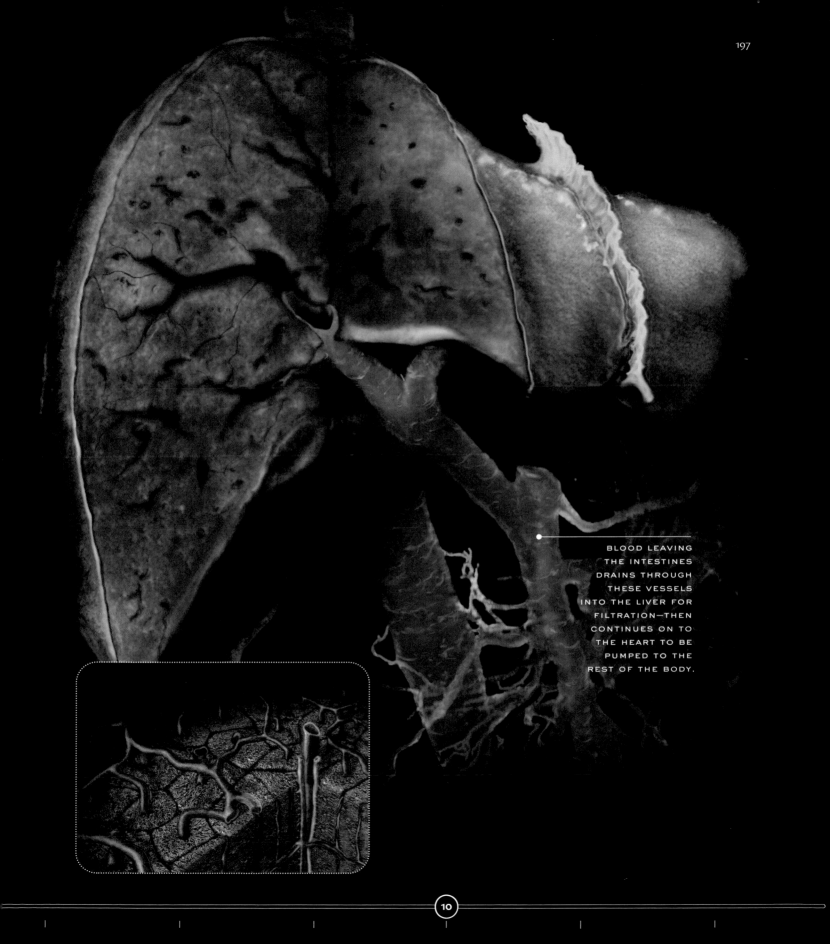

BLOOD LEAVING
THE INTESTINES
DRAINS THROUGH
THESE VESSELS
INTO THE LIVER FOR
FILTRATION—THEN
CONTINUES ON TO
THE HEART TO BE
PUMPED TO THE
REST OF THE BODY.

DUAL SYNTHESIZER

"In structure," according to *Gray's Anatomy*, published in 1901, "the pancreas resembles the salivary glands" but is "looser and softer in its texture."

Two organs in one, the pancreas secretes a battery of enzymes that together reduce digestible macromolecules into forms that the body can absorb. It also makes powerful hormones—chemical master switches—that govern the digestion of sugar, the most basic of fuels, and several other functions. Like the liver, its basic framework consists of lobules interspersed with branching blood, nerve, and drainage systems.

What's different, and what accounts for its more porous quality, is the predominance of 2 different cell types. The 98 percent of pancreatic cells that make enzymes are arranged in grapelike clusters: their secretions flow into larger and larger ducts, which eventually coalesce into the main pancreatic duct, which fuses with the main bile duct just before connecting to the duodenum. The other 2 percent—1 million or so column-shaped cell clusters that produce insulin and other hormones—are embedded like raisins in a cake, and drain through separate vessels into the bloodstream.

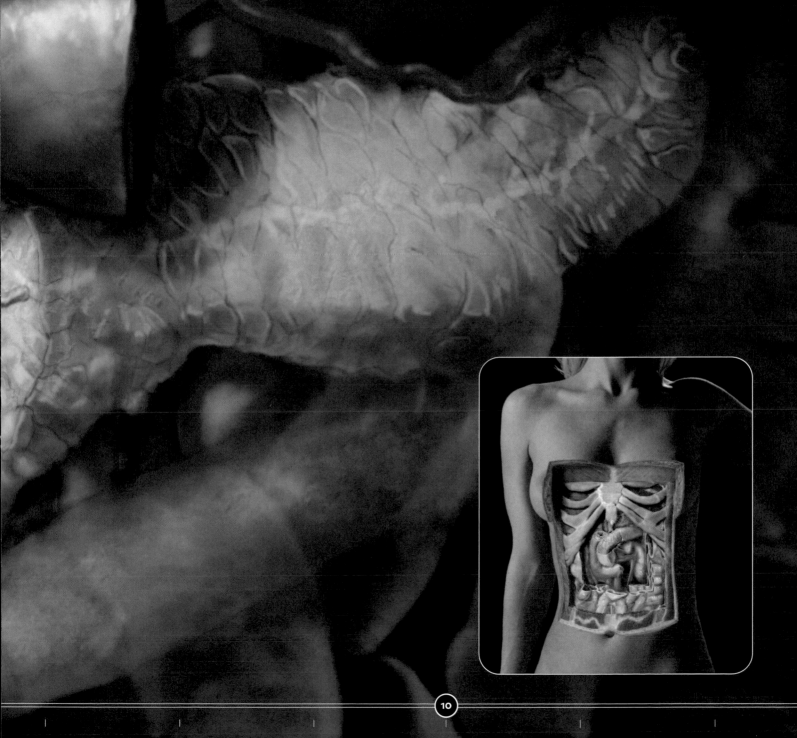

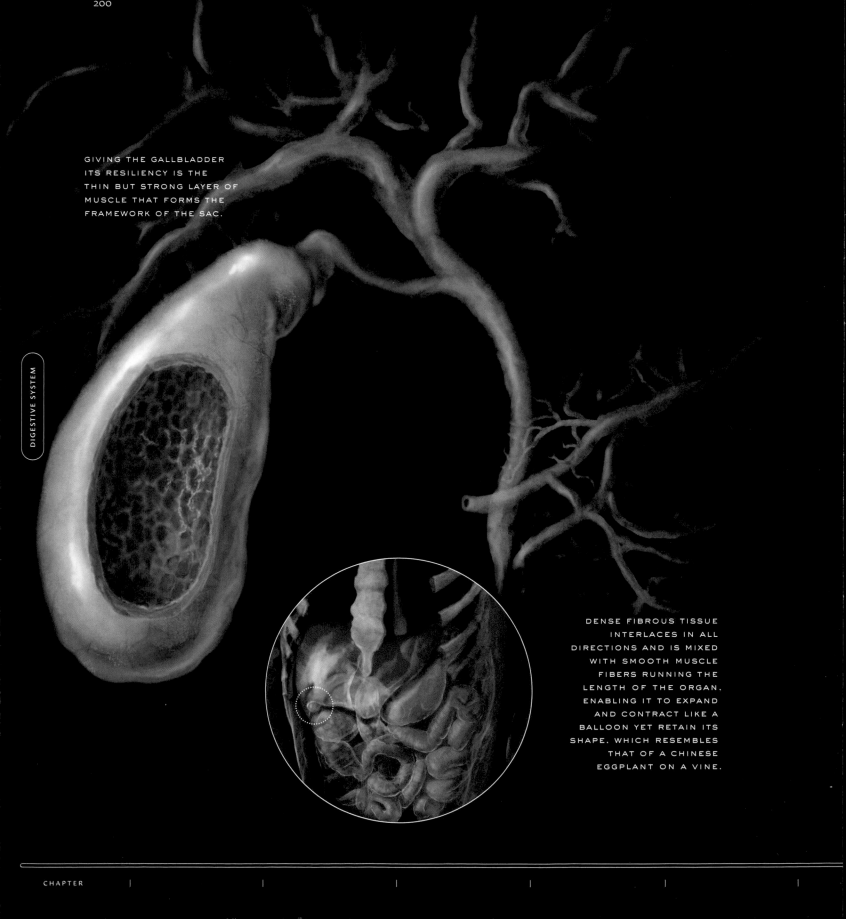

GIVING THE GALLBLADDER
ITS RESILIENCY IS THE
THIN BUT STRONG LAYER OF
MUSCLE THAT FORMS THE
FRAMEWORK OF THE SAC.

DIGESTIVE SYSTEM

DENSE FIBROUS TISSUE
INTERLACES IN ALL
DIRECTIONS AND IS MIXED
WITH SMOOTH MUSCLE
FIBERS RUNNING THE
LENGTH OF THE ORGAN,
ENABLING IT TO EXPAND
AND CONTRACT LIKE A
BALLOON YET RETAIN ITS
SHAPE, WHICH RESEMBLES
THAT OF A CHINESE
EGGPLANT ON A VINE.

One of the few organs whose name states its function, the gallbladder is a reservoir for a bitter substance. A soft, stretchy bag about 4 inches long and 1 inch wide at its thickest point, it collects bile, a thick yellow or greenish emulsion that turns fats into small droplets for easier digestion, much like detergents dissolve cooking grease. Its inner lining is crisscrossed by folds that absorb water from the bile, concentrating it by as much as 10 times before releasing it through a 2-way duct that maintains storage levels.

STORAGE

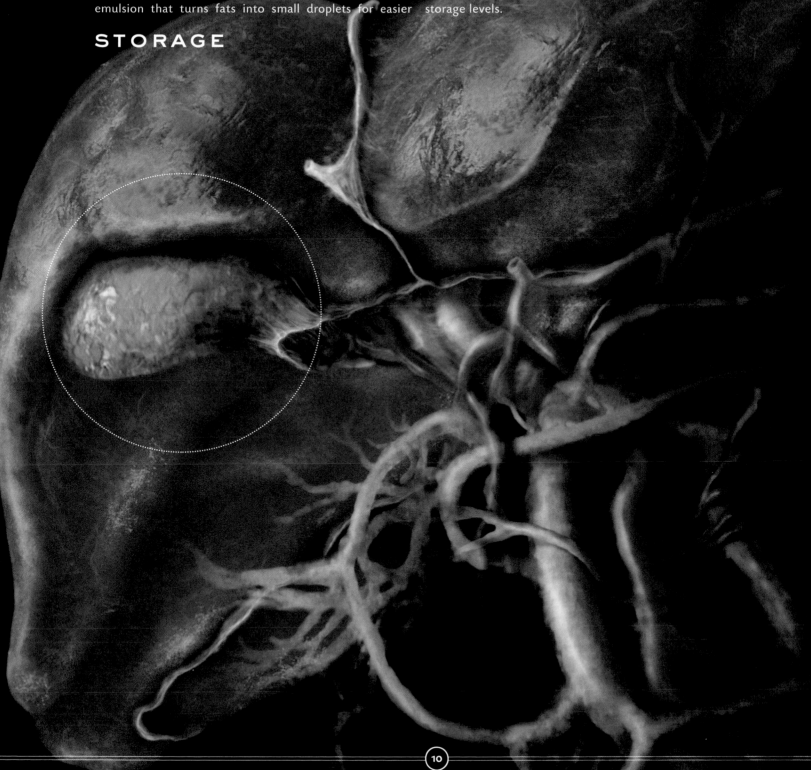

You're chyme. The trip down the gullet and through the stomach has churned you into tiny bits of organic nutrients, but now you face a *transforming event*—absorption.

The small intestine is an absorption system par excellence disguised as a coiled snake. You enter at the organ's mouth, where pancreatic juice and bile turn you into warm slush. The wall of the small intestine has an outer layer of longitudinal muscle surrounding an inner layer of circular muscle, and as the longitudinal muscle contracts involuntarily, the circular muscle just ahead of you relaxes. This makes the cavity wider, allowing more of you through.

The pulsing causes you to swirl, and as you swirl you hit the inner wall. Folds extending like circular shelves give the wall a corrugated texture and increase the surface area. But the greatest boost to surface area are from the millions of waving, tightly packed, fingerlike projections, villi (RIGHT) that stick

ABSORPTION

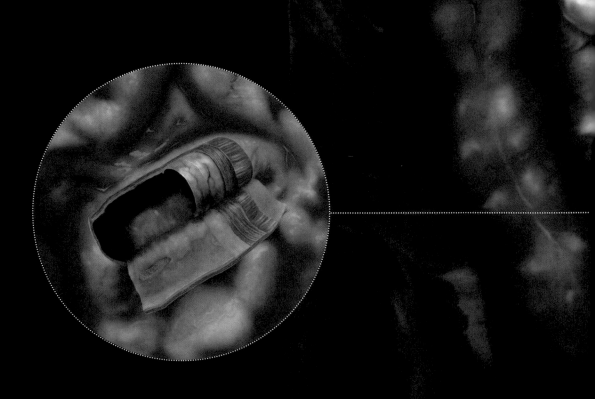

inward from the lining. These in turn are coated with microscopic "brush borders"—chemical countertops fastened with enzymes. It's this "fuzzy coat" that breaks the last string, snatching your molecules and whisking them inside the villi, where blood and lymph vessels ferry them away to the rest of the body. Blood vessels take the nutrient-rich blood from the small intestines and transport it to the liver for filtering (A, B, AND C) before traveling to nourish the rest of the body.

In less than 2 hours, 95 percent of your fats and 90 percent of your protein components are taken; all that's left is water and slag. If further measures of efficiency are necessary, it's estimated that if the small intestine had a smooth inner surface it would need to be more than 2 miles long, and that without the lightninglike power of enzymes to speed the process along, an average meal would require 6 months to digest.

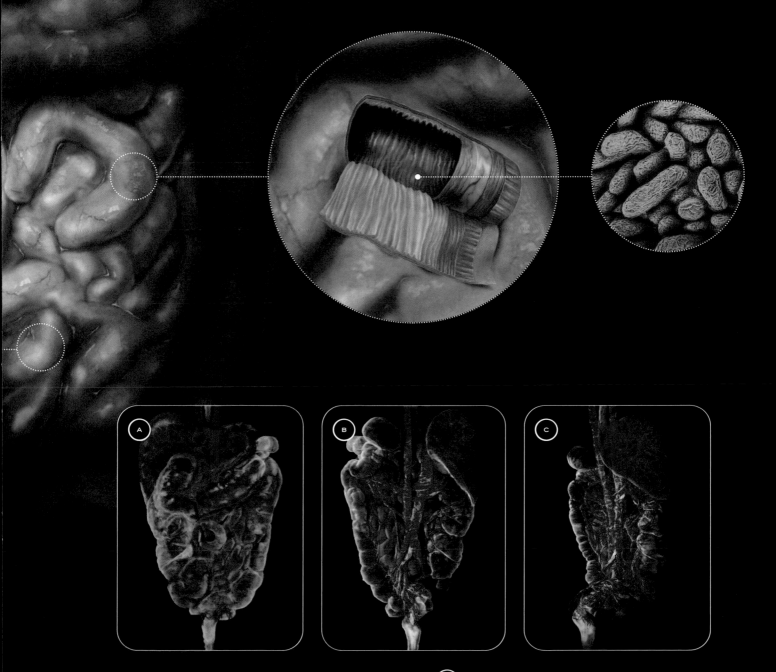

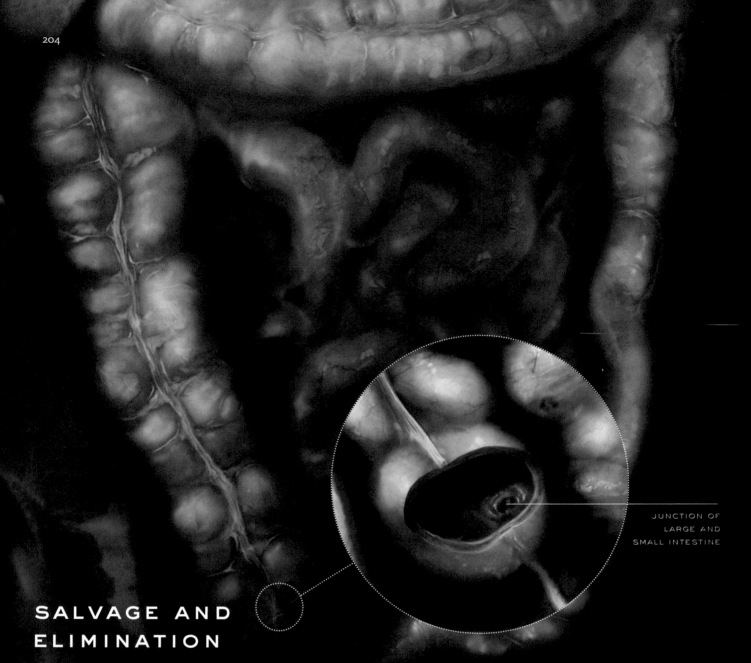

JUNCTION OF
LARGE AND
SMALL INTESTINE

SALVAGE AND
ELIMINATION

Arched illustriously over the small intestine like the edge of a shield, the bowel's job is to reduce, solidify, and eliminate the waste stream coming from the digestive tract—a combination trash compactor and composter. Since most of the volume of human waste is water, the inner lining is coated with water-absorbing cells. About 20 pints of water per day are needed to move food and nutrients through the alimentary canal, but almost all of it is eventually reabsorbed, so that the body doesn't become dehydrated. Meanwhile, muscle bands cinch and gather the colon into a series of pockets that help compact waste before passing it on.

The last stages of digestion are accomplished not by the body but by resident microbes. There are more bacteria in the warm, moist interior of the large intestine than throughout the rest of the body—so many that they form up to a 1-inch coating. Their job is to break down organic matter—manufacturing in the process useful chemicals such as Vitamin K that are absorbed back into the blood—and to produce gas. The final, necessary product of digestion is feces, an amalgam of water, undigested fiber, dead gut cells, living and dead bacteria (50 percent of the fecal mass), and digested bile pigments, which give them their color.

Bowel movements begin involuntarily but end, thanks to the ringlike outer sphincter of the anus, within our control—like swallowing in reverse.

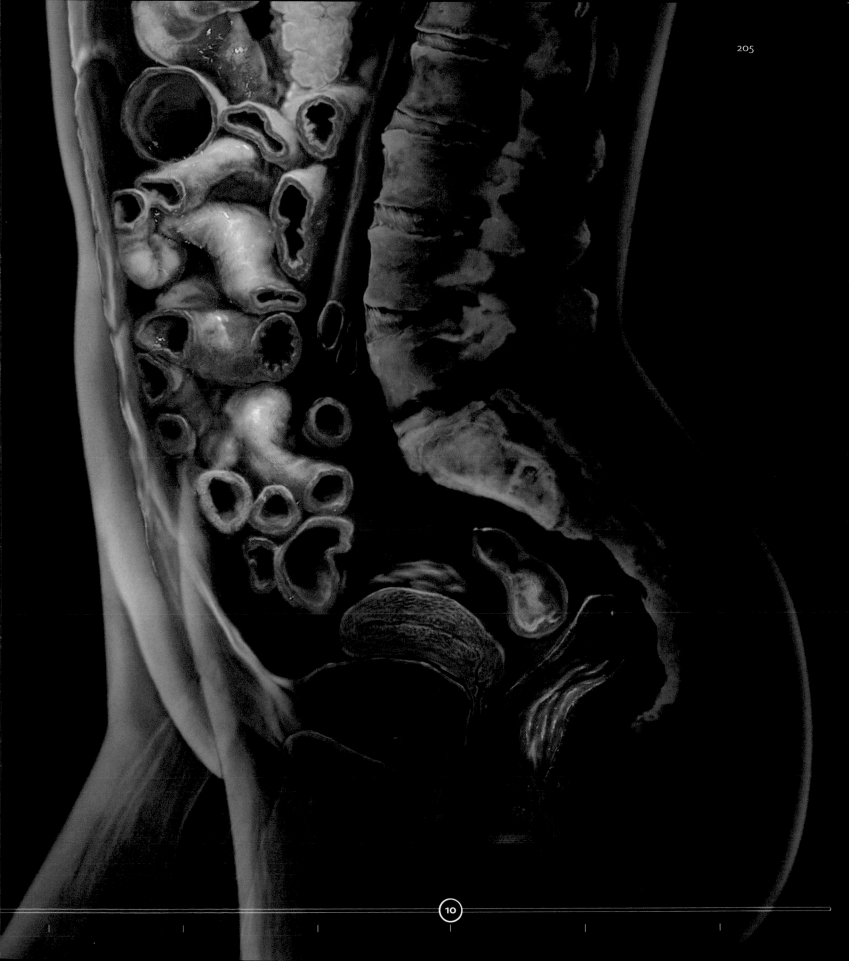

Microscopic structures in the mouth contribute to our pleasure in eating, which involves not only flavor but also what food scientists call "mouthfeel," the tactile sensation of food as it is being chewed. Onion-shaped taste buds (A) are located within the tiny mounds that give the tongue its velvety texture, which themselves are named for organic shapes: *fungiform* ("mushroomlike") on the front of the tongue, *circumvallate* ("ring-like") in the rear, and *foliate* ("leaflike") in the small trenches on the sides. Cells that pump out liquid for saliva are similarly orb-shaped (B),

some looking like half-moons against others and thus called *demilunes.*

Heavier and harder than most types of bone, the dense, mineral-laced network of cells inside our teeth (C) acts like a "crumple-resistant scaffolding," according to the *Encyclopedia of the Human Body*, edited by Richard Walker, "transmitting the force of the bite between the crown and the jaw." Further on, in the lining of the esophagus, seen here, cilial cells (D) stroke an overlying layer of mucus like tiny oars, moving in an arclike manner to lubricate the flow of food.

FUNCTIONAL UNITS (UPPER TRACT)

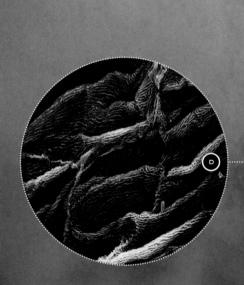

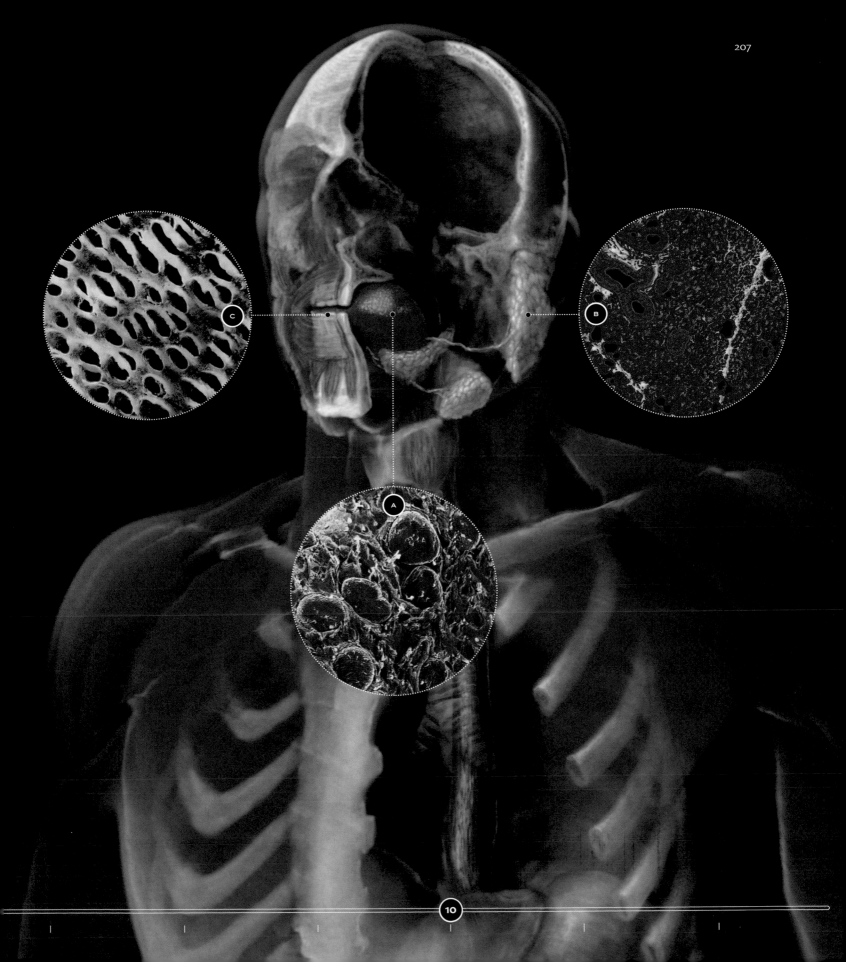

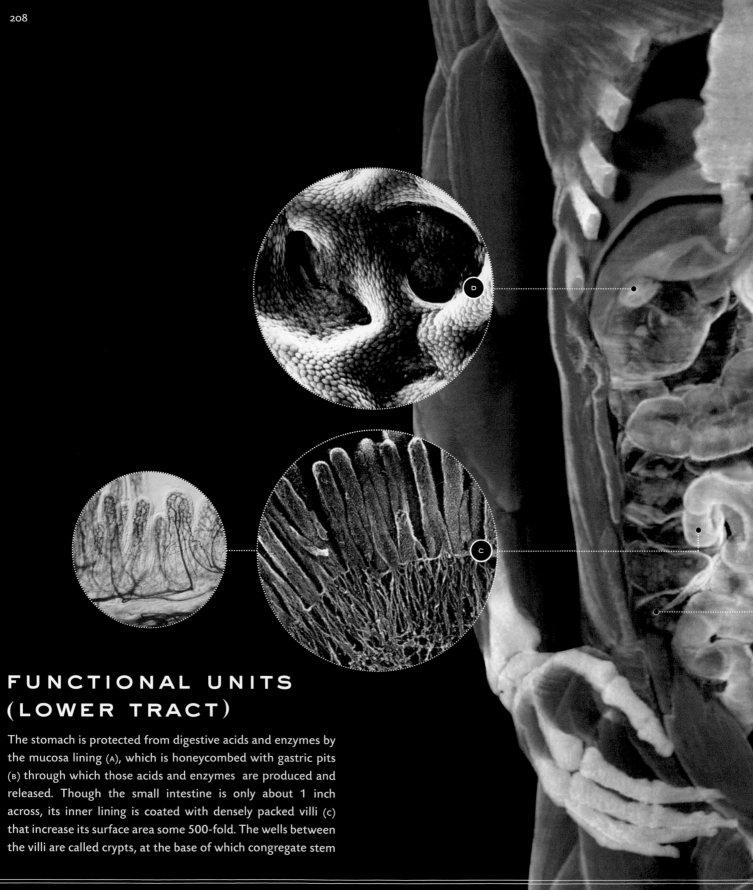

FUNCTIONAL UNITS (LOWER TRACT)

The stomach is protected from digestive acids and enzymes by the mucosa lining (A), which is honeycombed with gastric pits (B) through which those acids and enzymes are produced and released. Though the small intestine is only about 1 inch across, its inner lining is coated with densely packed villi (C) that increase its surface area some 500-fold. The wells between the villi are called crypts, at the base of which congregate stem

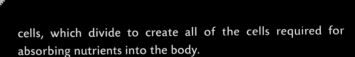

cells, which divide to create all of the cells required for absorbing nutrients into the body.

Throughout the lower gastrointestinal tract, cells work to absorb the copious amounts of water previously needed for digestion. Folds crisscrossing the lining of the gallbladder (D) remove water from bile, concentrating its fat-dissolving enzymes, while in the colon (E) puckered openings lead to tubular glands that draw water from feces.

MIRRORED IN NATURE

When nature develops a successful way of solving a problem, it doesn't throw it away. For instance, since the design problem of maximizing surface area is universal, it simply "replays" one of the many "tapes" in its library of optimal forms. Thus, the porous, crumple-proof lattice that makes teeth stronger than bone resembles the crush-resistant infrastructure of the stem of a buttercup.

DIGESTIVE SYSTEM

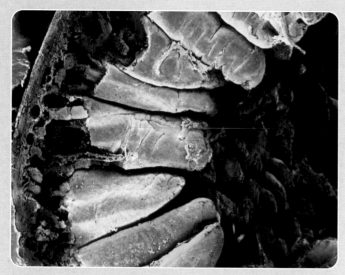

CROSS SECTION OF WALL OF SMALL INTESTINE

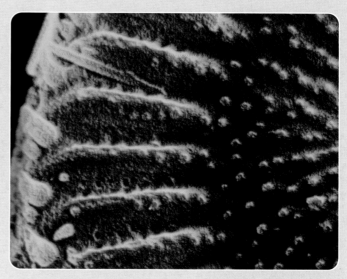

CYCLOTELLA MENEGHINIANA—A SINGLE-CELLED ALGAE

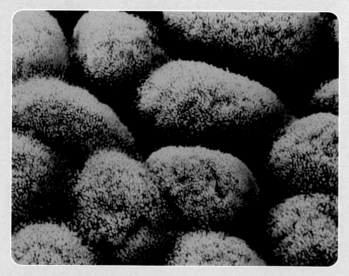

SURFACE CELLS OF GALLBLADDER

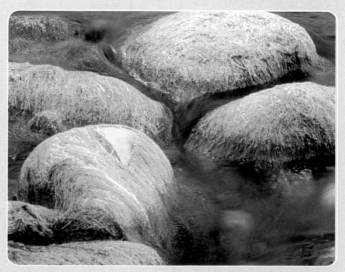

MOSS ALGAE ON ROCK SURFACE

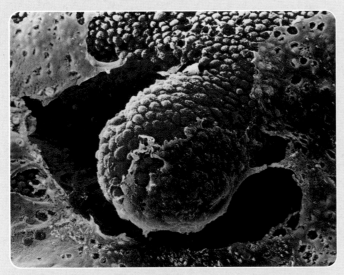

SURFACE CELLS OF COLON

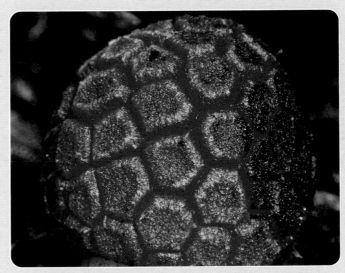

PARASITIC FLOWERING PLANT

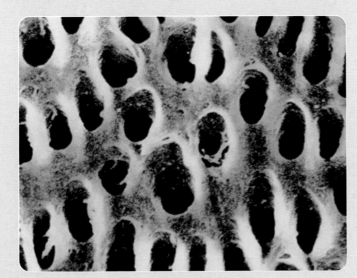

DENTAL TISSUE

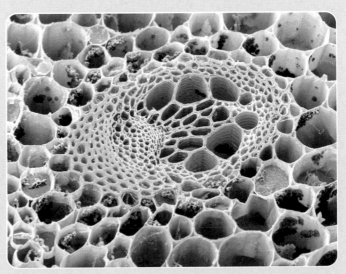

STEM OF A BUTTERCUP

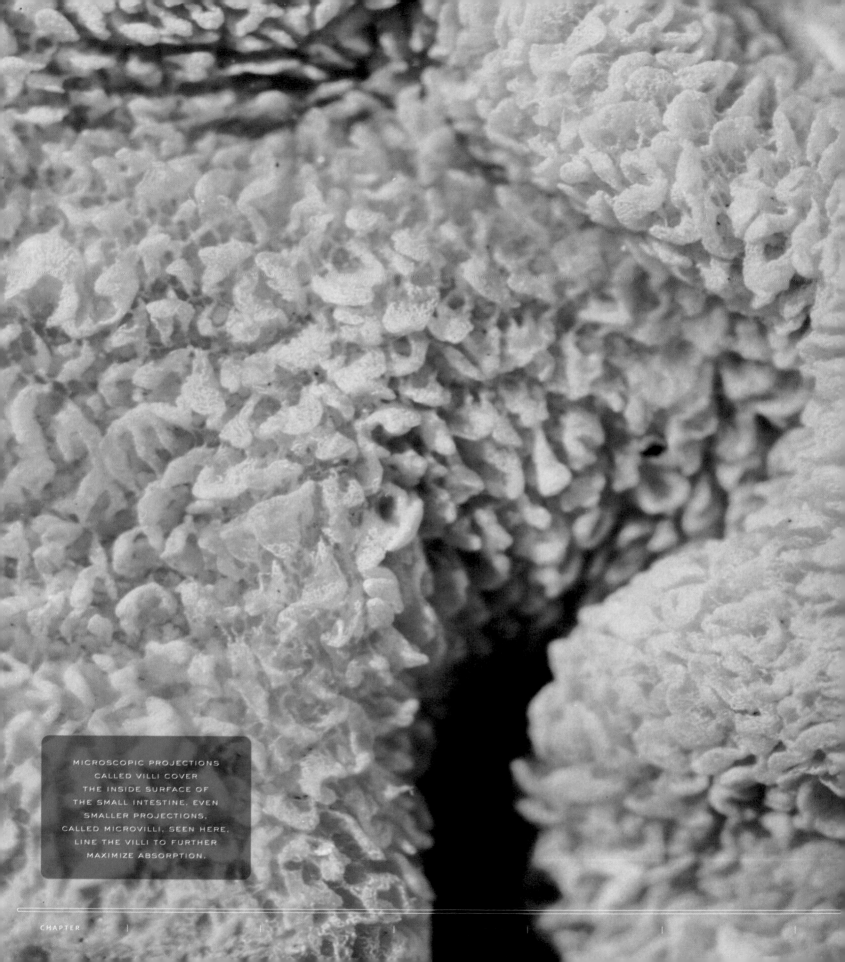

MICROSCOPIC PROJECTIONS
CALLED VILLI COVER
THE INSIDE SURFACE OF
THE SMALL INTESTINE. EVEN
SMALLER PROJECTIONS,
CALLED MICROVILLI, SEEN HERE,
LINE THE VILLI TO FURTHER
MAXIMIZE ABSORPTION.

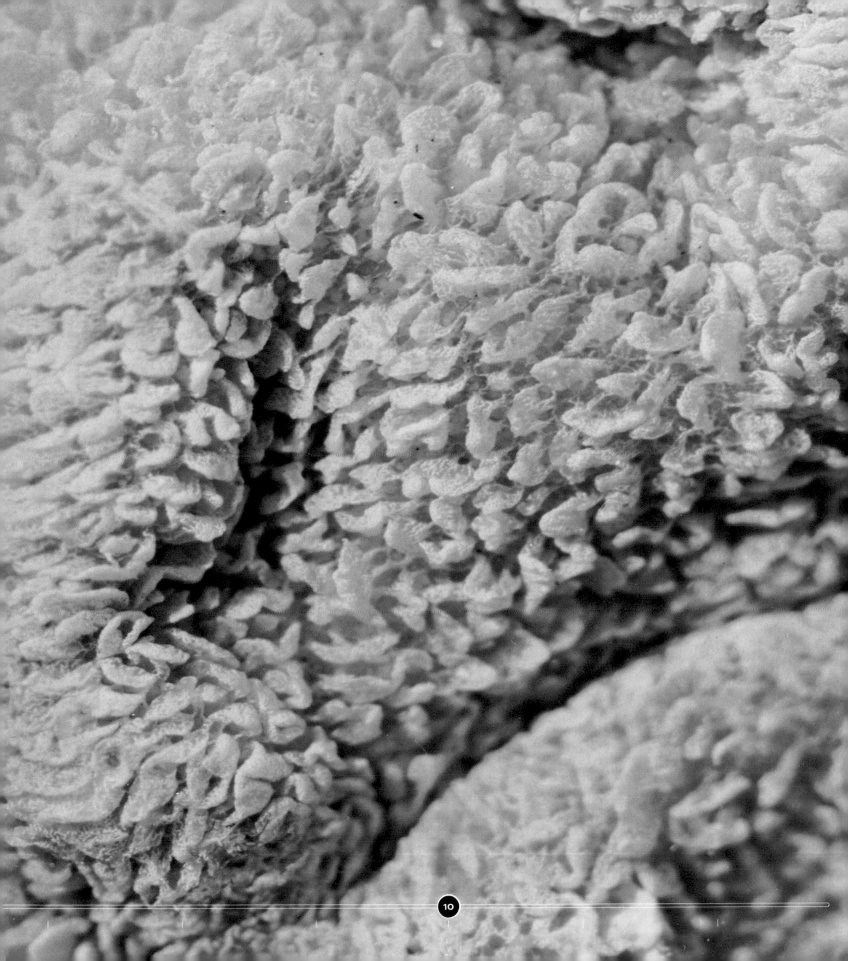

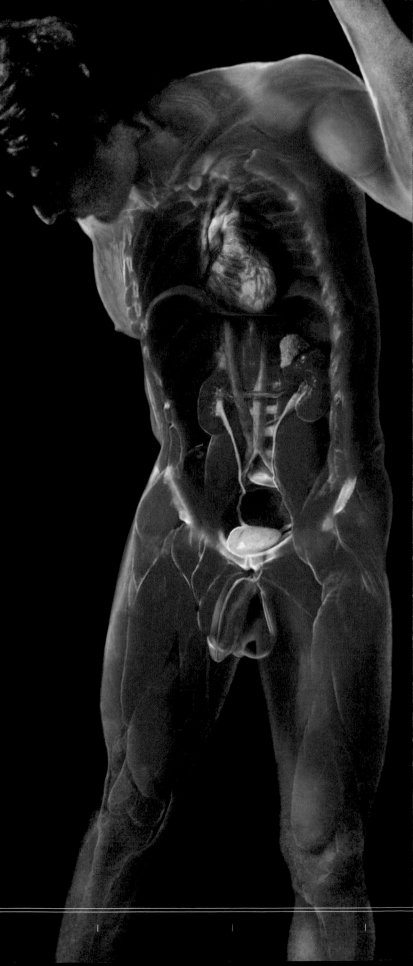

water and sewer

(urinary system)

The body is a water-in, water-out system, but unlike the lungs—our other chief exchange organ—the urinary apparatus doesn't simply take in, then strip apart vital materials. It also *recharges* them, adjusting their levels, balancing their presence in the blood. Central and secondary intakes and outflows are separated by an infrastructure of dams, reservoirs, sluices, valves, chemical treatment units, and feedback mechanisms. The scientific term for urination, *micturition*, means "making water," and urine isn't merely effluent. It's the outflow of some of the body's most advanced fluid and chemical engineering.

Water comprises 60 percent of our adult weight and is concentrated not only in the blood but in tissues such as skeletal muscle that hold moisture. Water distributes heat,

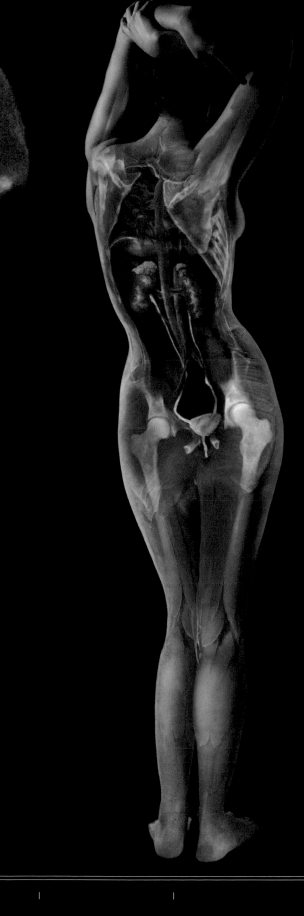

transports nutrients and hormones within and between cells, dilutes toxins, and serves as mother liquor for all chemical reactions. Yet we lose 2 quarts or more daily in exhaled breath, sweat, and feces, and if it becomes too salty or acidic, or too sweet, or contains too few red blood cells, we get sick. (Medieval physicians engaged in "urine gazing," inspecting and sometimes tasting urine to diagnose disease.) Mechanically speaking, the challenge of filtering microscopic wastes from 15 gallons of daily recirculating fluid while preserving pressure, volume, and compositional balance has yielded a 3-phase solution: accumulation, storage, and elimination. Men and women mainly differ, as women often lament, in the last phase, when anatomical variations are pronounced.

The work of protecting and regulating the fetal blood supply is outsourced, like back-office functions of Wall Street brokerages that are turned over to firms in Delhi. During pregnancy, fetal blood is cleaned and reconstituted in the placenta, even though unborn kidneys are functional by the fourth month. The mother's kidneys are forced to work overtime while her ballooning uterus presses harder and harder on her bladder, a spongelike holding tank, held back only by a short muscular tube one-fifth the length of a man's. No wonder she doesn't sleep. (She gets her revenge years later, when the enlarging prostates of the men throttle their urethras, causing similar problems.)

When the baby is born, the mother's kidneys are suddenly relieved of a load (her bladder will take longer to recover) just as the newborn's spring instantly into use. That babies often urinate within seconds after their umbilical cords are cut attests to the speed of the transfer.

FILTERING FOR TWO

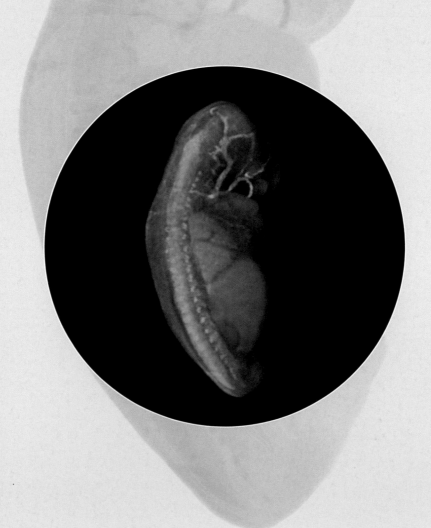

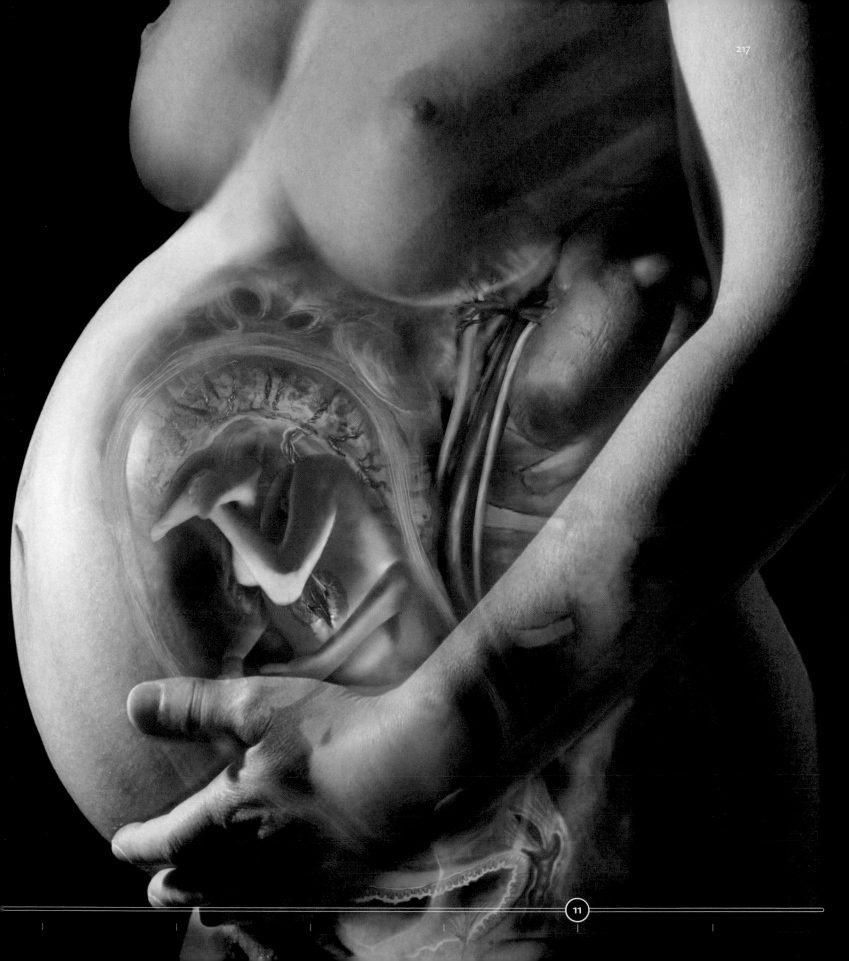

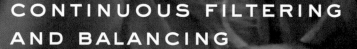

CONTINUOUS FILTERING AND BALANCING

Designers of filtration systems, especially in "wet" fields like dairy, blood, and water purification, exalt the kidneys. Two bean-shaped organs at the back of the abdominal cavity, each about the size of a fist, the kidneys comprise about one-twentieth of the body's weight, yet receive, with each heartbeat, one fifth of its blood—a rate of 45 gallons, or about 8 thorough cleanings, per day. Perfusing through a fan-shaped core consisting of pyramid-shaped masses, the blood is separated and reconstituted, and revitalized. Its wastes, excess water and salts, drain into a funnel-shaped cavity and out through a tube. Far more than a sluiceway for urine, the kidneys control blood homeostasis—they're the blood's brain and endocrine system, as well. When excesses are present, they're passed out through filtration, like a cappuccino maker where water is forced under pressure through a fine sieve. When the same substances are low, they're reclaimed through reabsorption, which, as biomedical writer Craig Freudenrich points out, is similar to the "fish pond game you see at some amusement parks" in which children try to catch different-colored fish magnets in a passing "stream." Like the children, so-called "transporters" catch and release key molecules in the filtrate, continuously regulating the blood's chemical balances within narrow limits.

Each kidney contains about 1 million functional units called nephrons, which resemble minuscule slide trombones ensnarled with coils. Combining the features of the cappuccino machine and the magnetic duck pond, the nephron's architecture includes a long thin tube encapsulating a thicket of capillaries at one end, 2 twisted regions interspaced with a long hairpin loop, and a long straight portion entwined by another thatch of capillaries at the other. The blood enters under pressure through the capsule, forming a filtrate, which, as it descends and ascends the loop, loses and picks up materials until it is chemically rebalanced and refreshed. Chemical feedback loops control the process. Much of the water and some salts and sugars are reabsorbed during filtration by surrounding veins and arteries.

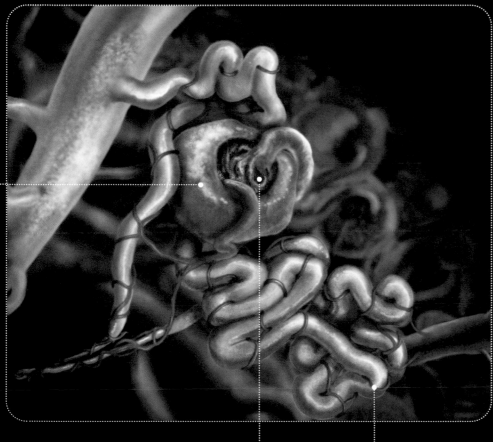

THE REMAINING SALTS, SUGARS, AND WATER COMPOSE THE WASTE THAT LEAVES EACH NEPHRON THROUGH A COLLECTING TUBULE TO TRAVEL TO THE URINARY BLADDER.

WASTE AND WATER ARE FIRST FILTERED HERE IN THE GLOMERULUS—A HIGH-PRESSURE CAPILLARY BED.

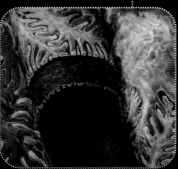
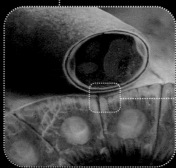
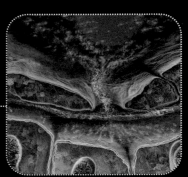

Layers of relaxed smooth muscle in the bladder wall encapsulate a folded inner lining. As the bladder swells with urine, the muscles stretch, causing the folds to iron out and disappear. Nerve receptors in the wall relay the extent of the stretching to the brain, which signals the desire to relax 2 ringlike sphincters—muscular spigots. The bladder's expandability is prodigious; though it can hold 200 to 300 milliliters (one-third to one-half a pint) before we have the urge to void, it's capable of ballooning to hold twice that much before we absolutely have to.

LIQUID TANKER

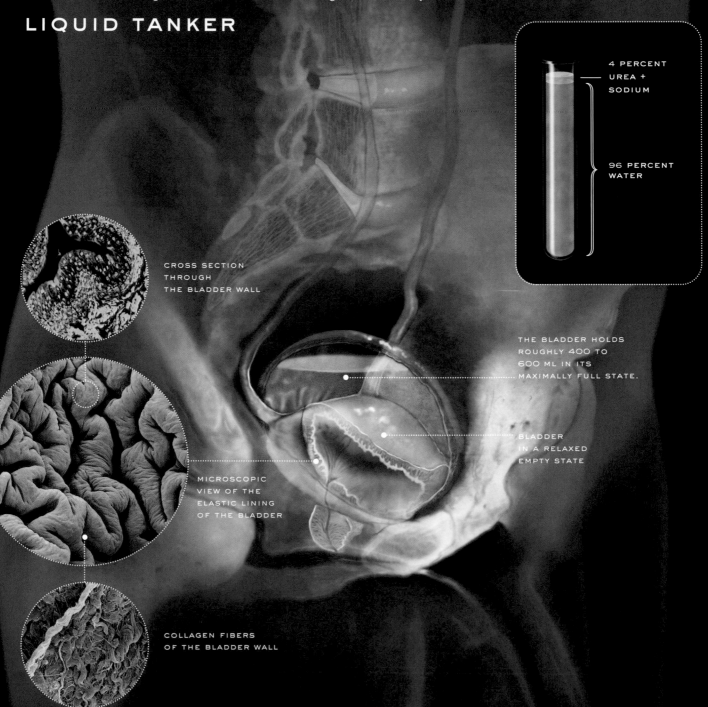

4 PERCENT
UREA +
SODIUM

96 PERCENT
WATER

CROSS SECTION
THROUGH
THE BLADDER WALL

THE BLADDER HOLDS
ROUGHLY 400 TO
600 ML IN ITS
MAXIMALLY FULL STATE.

BLADDER
IN A RELAXED
EMPTY STATE

MICROSCOPIC
VIEW OF THE
ELASTIC LINING
OF THE BLADDER

COLLAGEN FIBERS
OF THE BLADDER WALL

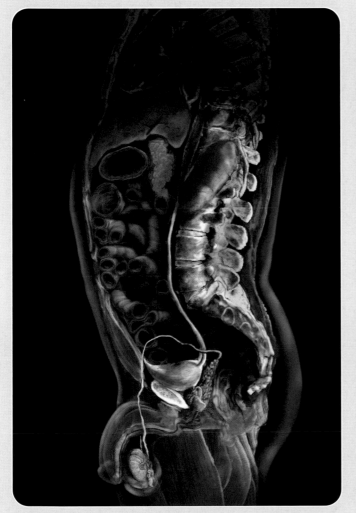

MAN

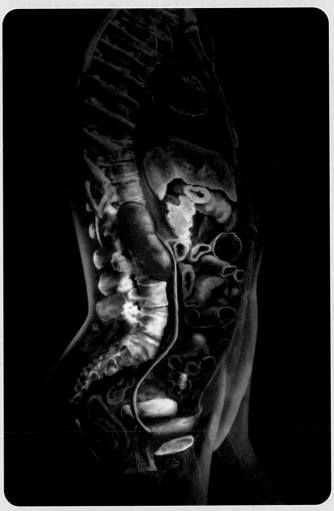

WOMAN

GENDER DIFFERENCES

Produced in a continuous trickle at a rate of about 1 milliliter per minute, urine is "milked" by two contracting tubes (ureters) that lead to the bladder, a highly stretchy holding tank crammed in the reproductive region. The physical (and social, and psychological) objective behind channeling and controlling urine flow beyond that point is to ensure a voluntary, if not always sanitary or convenient, release. "In France one must adapt oneself to the fragrance of the urinal," Gertrude Stein noted, adding that "the Parisians are all wine drinkers and for a gentleman the bladder is more restless than for a lady."

MIRRORED IN NATURE

The structures of the urinary tract, all involved with fluid management, employ motifs from other natural realms whose purposes are often quite different. Braided collagen fibers that stretch to expand the bladder wall resemble moth antennae, which are sensitive chemoreceptors, combing out pheromones from the opposite sex. The membranous folds of tissue that disappear

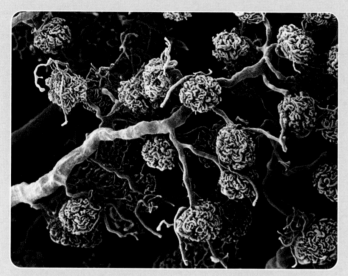

KIDNEY BLOOD VESSELS

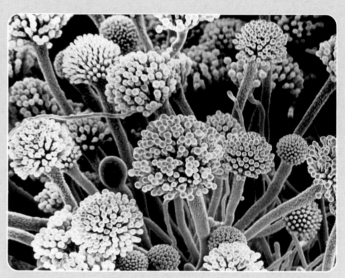

ASPERGILLUS FUNGUS

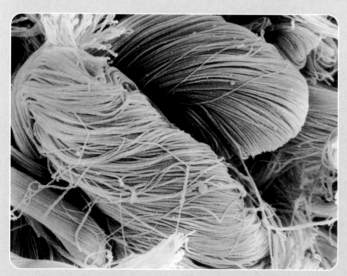

COLLAGEN FIBERS OF BLADDER

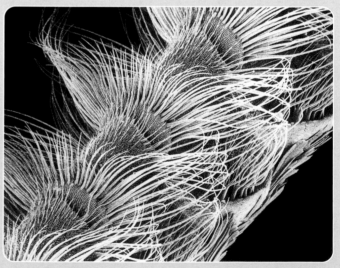

MOTH ANTENNAE

when the bladder stretches look like the hymenal undersides of mushrooms, which produce spores. Kidney blood vessels, interlaced with nephrons, and kidney tubules, which collect urine, share similarities with, respectively, aspergillus spores (common fungi that grow on decaying vegetation and cause lung spasms in many allergy sufferers) and sea anemone tentacles (which snare food).

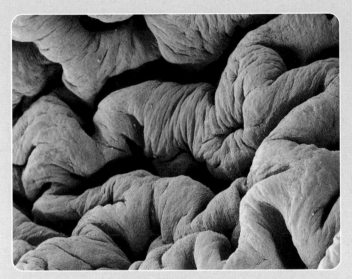

BLADDER WALL

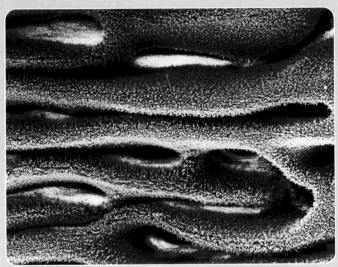

MUSHROOM GILLS

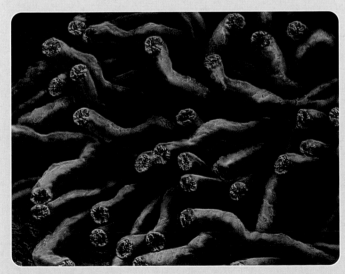

KIDNEY TUBULES

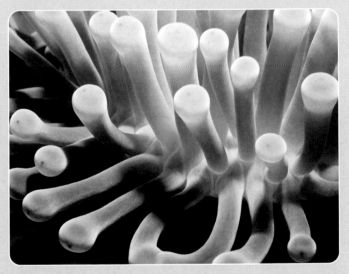

SEA ANEMONE TENTACLES

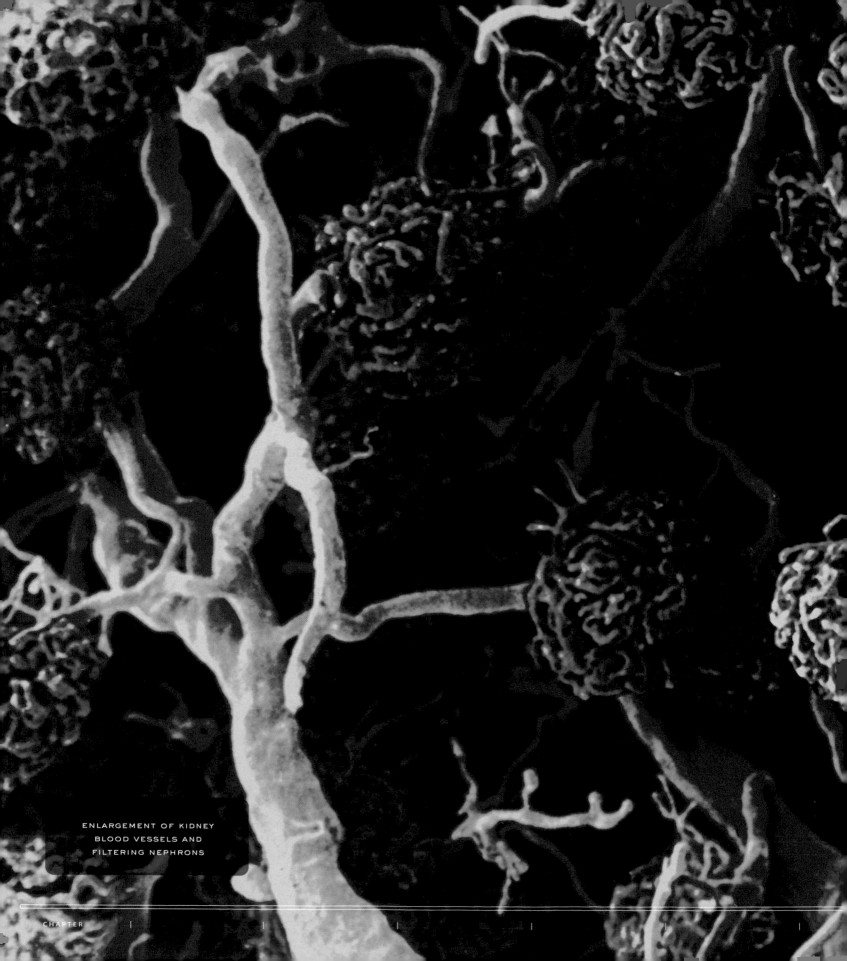

ENLARGEMENT OF KIDNEY
BLOOD VESSELS AND
FILTERING NEPHRONS

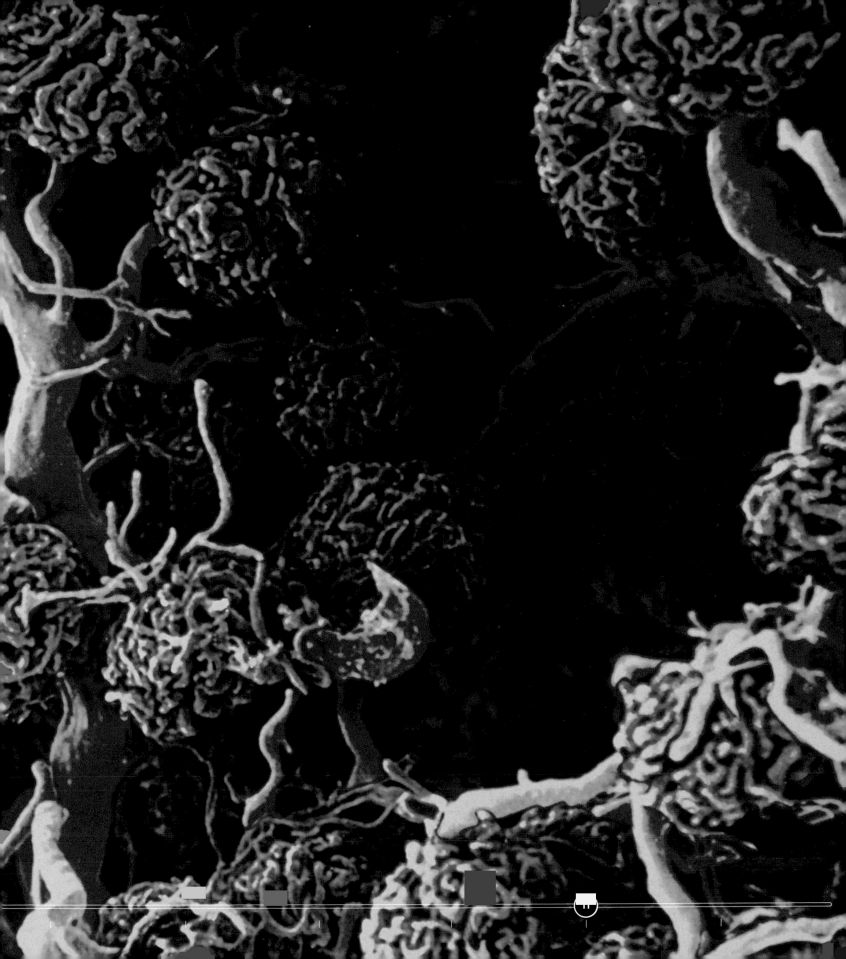

Sex is something I really don't understand too hot . . .
I keep making up these sex rules for myself, and
then break them right away.
—Holden Caulfield, *The Catcher in the Rye*

replication

(reproductive system)

It's not only teenage virgins who are confounded by sexual reproduction. Comedian Marty Feldman said, "Sex is two and two makes five" and aphorist Mason Cooley describes it as "not imaginary, but it's not quite real either." British author Anne Cumming called sex "a shortcut to everything"; John Dos Passos, "a slot machine"; gay wit Quentin Crisp, "the last refuge of the miserable"; Henry Miller, "one of the nine reasons for reincarnation—the other eight are unimportant." John Updike says, "Sex is like money, only too much is enough," while social critic Camille Paglia responds, "Sex is metaphysical for men, as it is not for women. Women have no problem to solve through sex."

The problem solved through sex could not be more universal or key—the imperative for species and individuals to replicate—yet men and women disagree, often radically, about its meanings. This dispute can be both needed and desirable, since sex, as Peter Ustinov observed, "is a conversation carried out through other means." But the fact that we confer sexuality and the mechanisms of sexual behavior with meaning at all is perhaps what gives them their greatest power and mystery, and invites so many contradictory attempts to have the last word. "Sex is," Gore Vidal summarized tersely. "There is nothing more to be done about it. Sex builds no roads, writes no novels, and sex certainly gives no meaning to anything in life but itself."

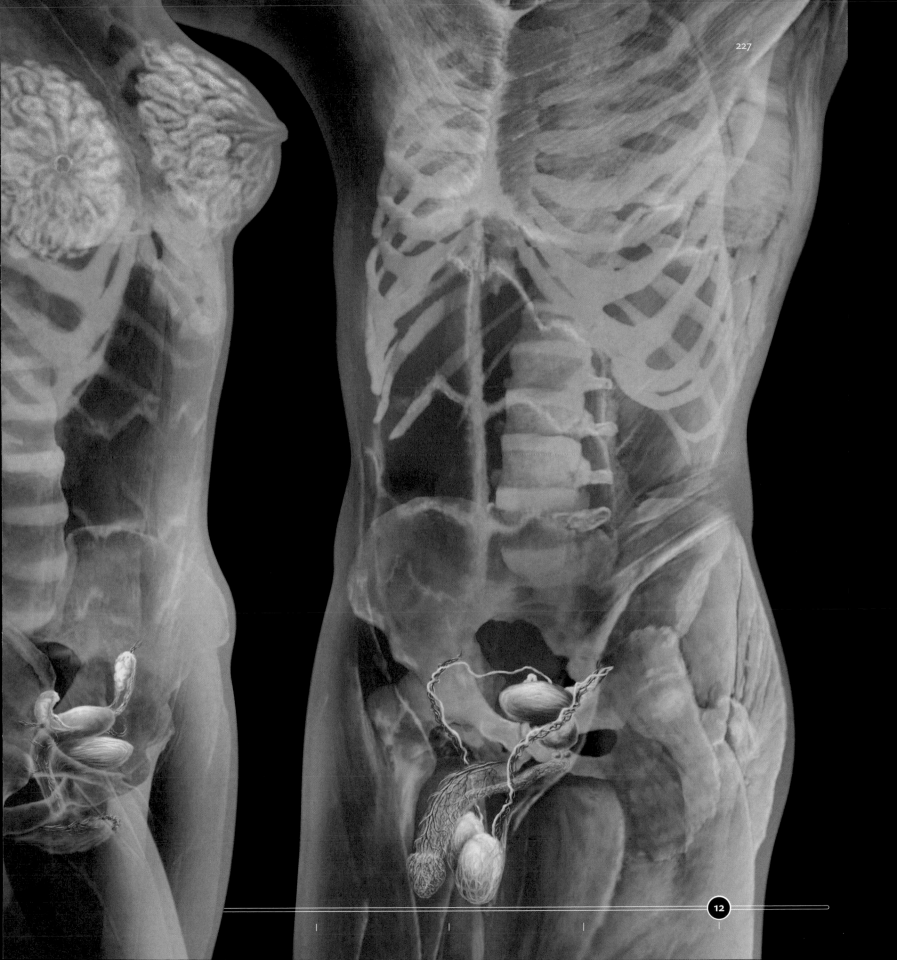

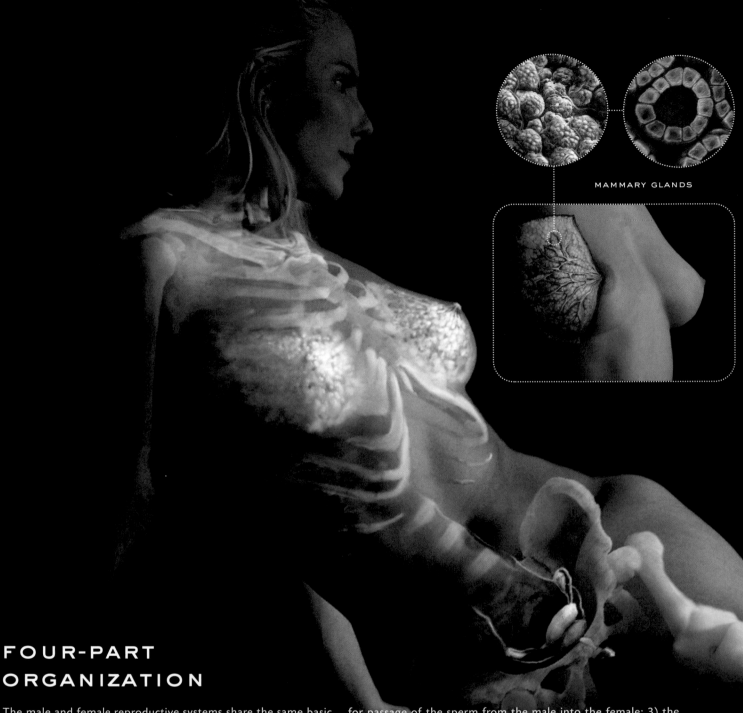

MAMMARY GLANDS

FOUR-PART ORGANIZATION

The male and female reproductive systems share the same basic 4-part organization: 1) the gonads (ovaries or testes) produce special reproductive cells (eggs or sperm), which carry half the normal chromosomal contingent of other cells in the body and unite during fertilization; gonads also carry steroid hormones essential for reproduction, bodily growth, and development; 2) the genitals (penis in males, clitoris and vulva in females) allow for passage of the sperm from the male into the female; 3) the ducts and accessory glands connect the gonads to the genitals, forming a kind of ecosystem in which final preparations for fertilization are made and the resulting embryo is nurtured; and 4) a 2-tiered feedback network ties the gonads to the hypothalamus and other endocrine structures in order to regulate the secretion of the steroid hormones.

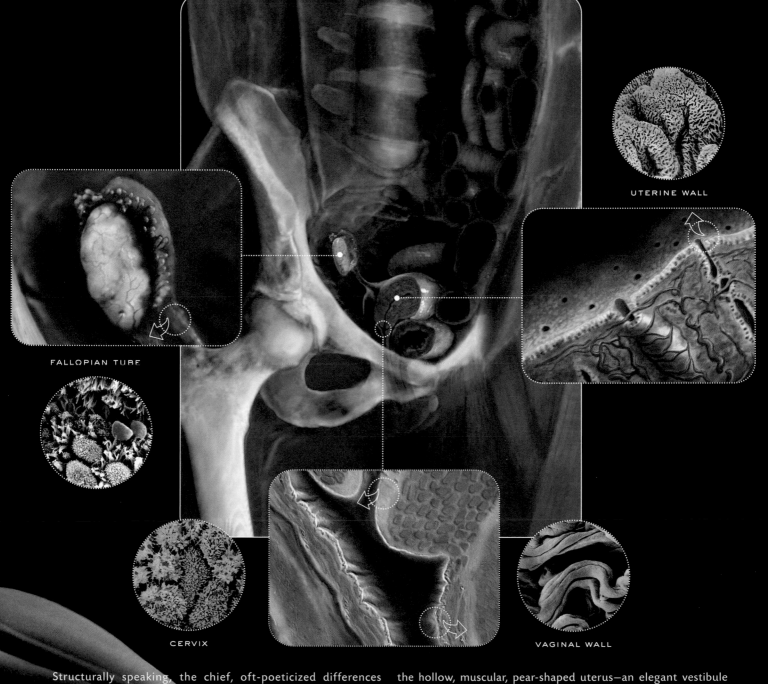

UTERINE WALL

FALLOPIAN TUBE

CERVIX

VAGINAL WALL

Structurally speaking, the chief, oft-poeticized differences between the sexes stem from the expanded role, in women, of the ducts and accessory organs—the vagina, uterus, and breasts. Built of skin, muscle, and fibrous tissue and lined with a lubricating membrane, the vagina is a 4-to-5-inch tunnel extending from the outer opening to a donut-shaped ring of muscles that guards the hollow, muscular, pear-shaped uterus—an elegant vestibule to the embryo containment area at the heart of the apparatus. Clusters of mammary glands in the breasts are made up of lobes and lobules that secrete milk into 15 to 20 tubelike ducts, each discharging through a tiny separate orifice in the nipple.

230

Of all the body's cells, the mature ovum alone is spherical. "The shape makes sense," science writer Natalie Angier notes. "A sphere is one of the most stable shapes in nature. If you want to protect your most sacred heirlooms—your genes—bury them in spherical treasure chests."

Six to seven million immature eggs are produced during gestation, with all but 40,000 or so destroyed naturally before puberty. From then on, once a month, a potential crop of 15 to 20 are selected to begin maturation. A wave of hormones released from the pituitary washes over the pods, or follicles, in the ovaries where they're stored.

CYCLICAL
OPPORTUNITIES

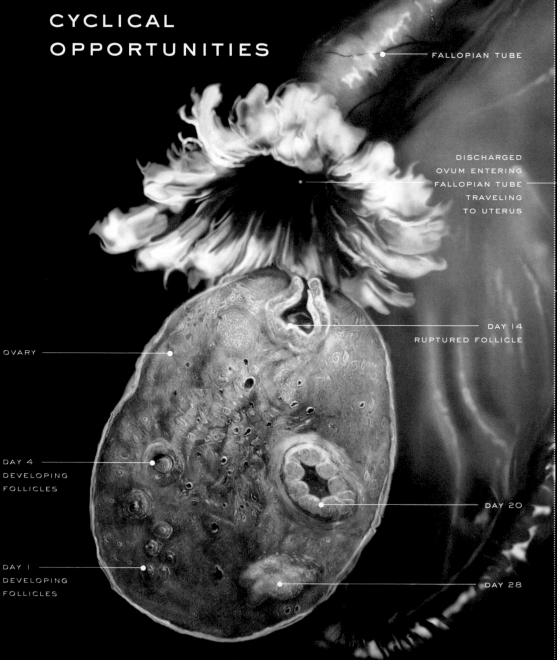

REPRODUCTIVE SYSTEM

FALLOPIAN TUBE

DISCHARGED
OVUM ENTERING
FALLOPIAN TUBE
TRAVELING
TO UTERUS

DAY 14
RUPTURED FOLLICLE

OVARY

DAY 4
DEVELOPING
FOLLICLES

DAY 20

DAY 1
DEVELOPING
FOLLICLES

DAY 28

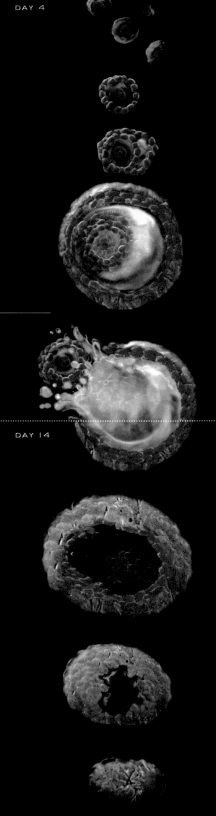

DAY 4

DAY 14

DAY 28

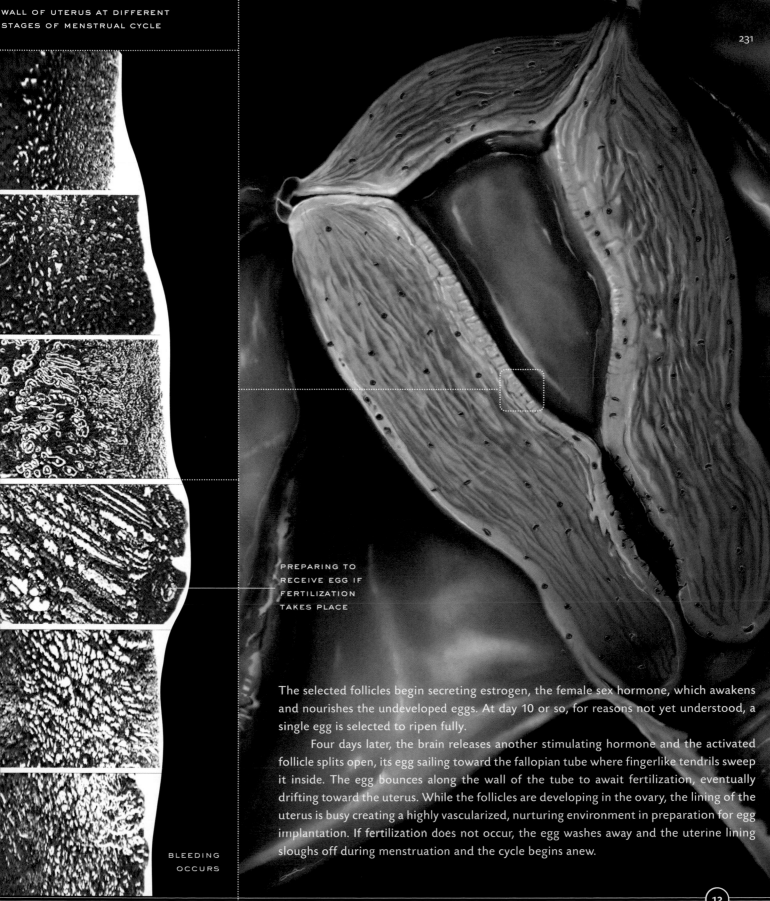

PREPARING TO
RECEIVE EGG IF
FERTILIZATION
TAKES PLACE

BLEEDING
OCCURS

The selected follicles begin secreting estrogen, the female sex hormone, which awakens and nourishes the undeveloped eggs. At day 10 or so, for reasons not yet understood, a single egg is selected to ripen fully.

Four days later, the brain releases another stimulating hormone and the activated follicle splits open, its egg sailing toward the fallopian tube where fingerlike tendrils sweep it inside. The egg bounces along the wall of the tube to await fertilization, eventually drifting toward the uterus. While the follicles are developing in the ovary, the lining of the uterus is busy creating a highly vascularized, nurturing environment in preparation for egg implantation. If fertilization does not occur, the egg washes away and the uterine lining sloughs off during menstruation and the cycle begins anew.

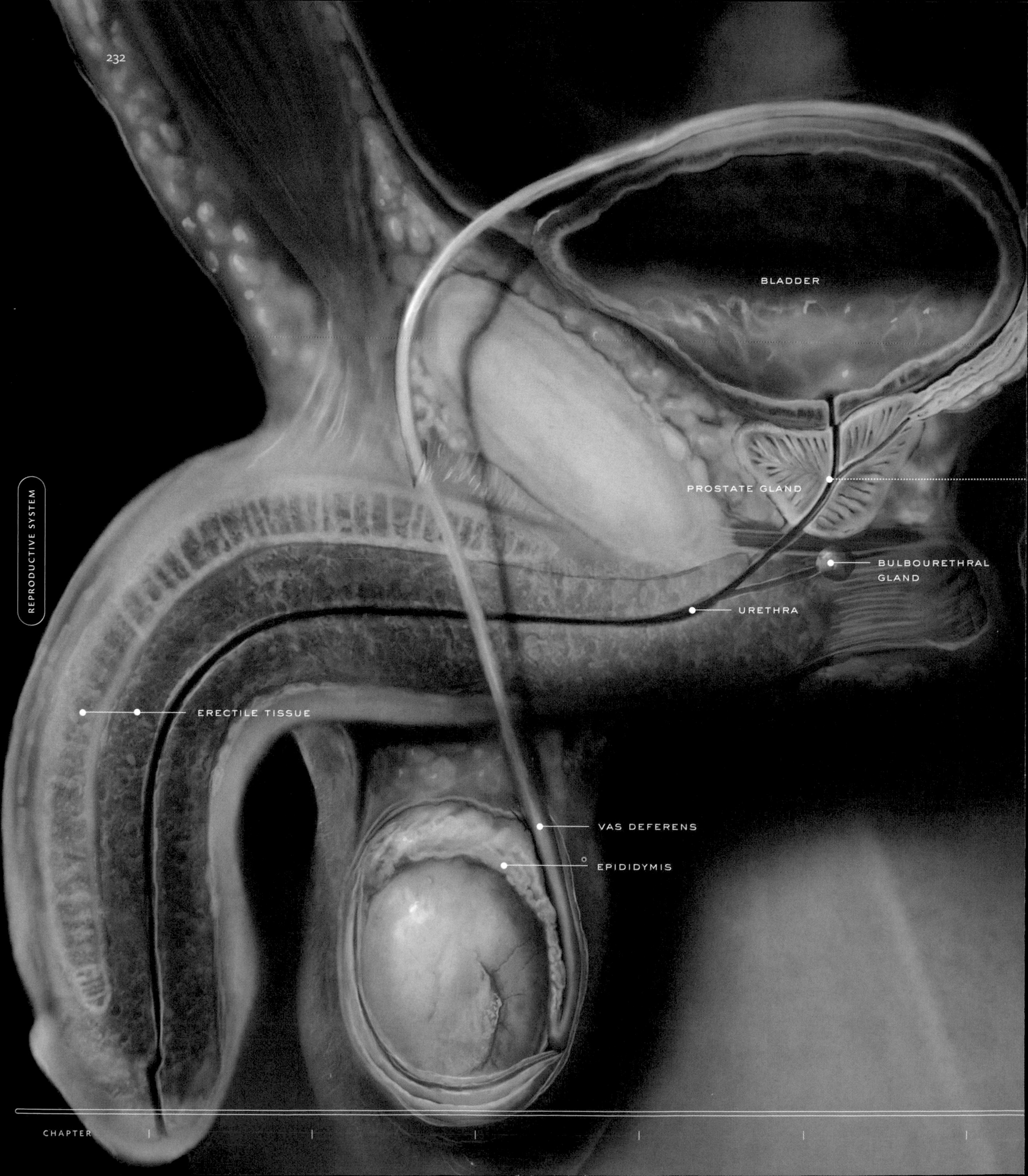

BLADDER

PROSTATE GLAND

BULBOURETHRAL
GLAND

URETHRA

ERECTILE TISSUE

VAS DEFERENS

EPIDIDYMIS

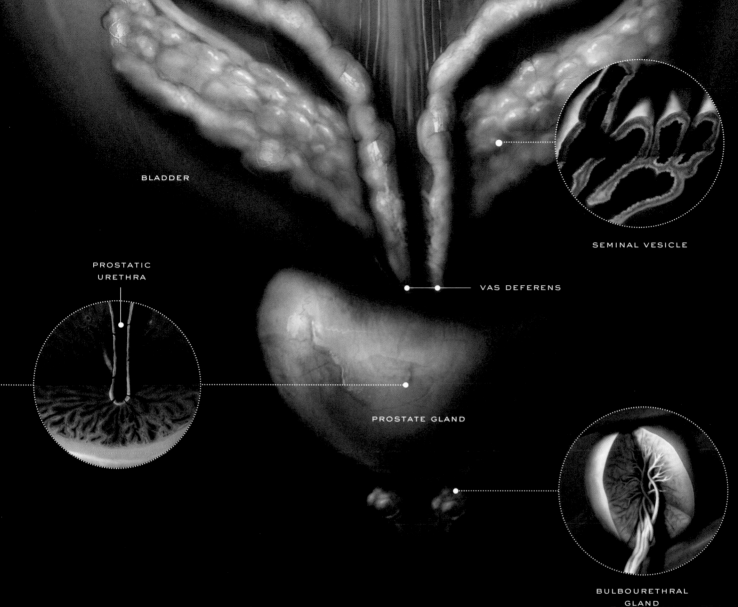

BLADDER

PROSTATIC
URETHRA

SEMINAL VESICLE

VAS DEFERENS

PROSTATE GLAND

BULBOURETHRAL
GLAND

LIQUID VESSEL
TRANSPORT

As a delivery service—a vector—for genetic material, the male sex organs are inspired by several needs: propulsion, lubrication, chemical balance, and sustenance of its cargo. Semen, the liquid vessel for transmitting genes to the nestled egg, is made up of sperm and the fluids that facilitate its movement. Up to 3,000 sperm per second (250 million per day) are produced in the testicles, 2 egg-shaped organs that hang just below the penis in the scrotum—outside the body wall for coolness (normal body temperatures are too warm for sperm production, but when the temperature outside is too cold, a thin layer of muscle surrounding the scrotum contracts to draw the testes closer to the body); the testicles

hang at slightly different altitudes, to keep them from jostling each other during ordinary movement. The sperm are stored in highly coiled ducts (epididymides) atop the testes until ejaculation, when they're propelled through parallel ductworks where secretions from 3 sets of glands fortify them for transit: mucus, amino acids, and super-sweet fructose for energy from the seminal vesicles; alkaline enzymes, to neutralize the natural acidity of the vagina and help activate the sperm, from the prostate; and, from the bulbourethral glands, another fluid to help neutralize any remaining acidic urine in the urethra and buffer sperm from physical impact.

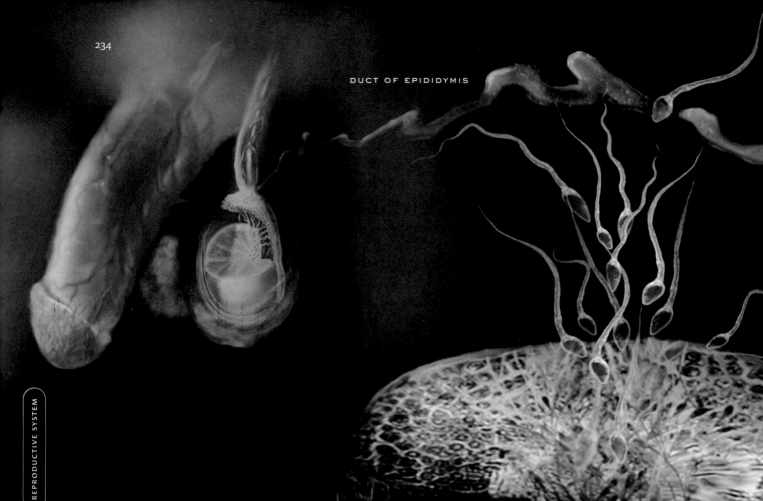

DUCT OF EPIDIDYMIS

SEMINIFEROUS
TUBULE

SEED CULTIVATION

A single testicle has about 300 compartments, each containing 1 to 4 tightly coiled tubules that, if unraveled, would stretch more than 5 football fields. The outer wall of these seminiferous tubules is packed from birth with unspecialized germ cells that, at puberty, begin dividing into sperm. Pressing inward as more and more develop, the sperm mature, their chromosomal complement halving as they migrate toward a central cavity that leads to the epididymis.

Designwise, the sperm is an uncommonly sleek vessel. Its ovoid head, enveloping the nucleus and its cargo of DNA, wears a protective cap containing an enzyme that helps the sperm penetrate the egg. Its braided midsection attaches head and tail and contains the power pack—mitochondria. Its whiplike tail tapers to a tasseled filament for added locomotion.

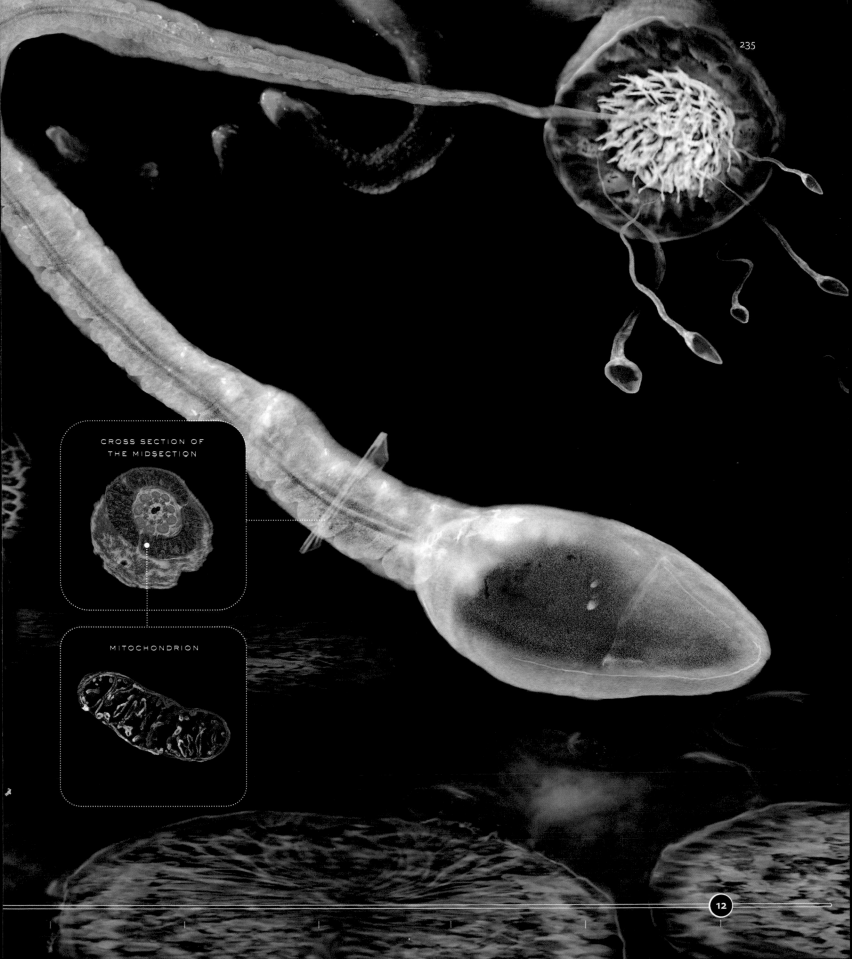

CROSS SECTION OF
THE MIDSECTION

MITOCHONDRION

The penis, novelist William Gass wrote, "is a ridiculous petitioner . . . It is so easily teased, insulted, betrayed, abandoned; yet it must pretend to be invulnerable, a weapon which confers magical powers on its possessor; consequently this muscleless inchworm must try to swagger through temples and pull apart thighs like the hairiest Sampson, the mightiest ram."

Passion and eroticism aside, male "performance" results mainly from 2 types of physics: hydraulics and bioelectrics. When a male is sexually aroused, the 3 panels of erectile tissue in his penis fill with blood; the organ becomes distended.

Once the blood is in place, the drainage vessels become compressed, slowing down blood outflow, prolonging erection. The penis is rafted with excitatory neurons, and when nerve impulses fired by further stimulation produce orgasm and ejaculation, drainage vessels open up again allowing it to return to a flaccid state. As a triple-purpose organ—eliminative, reproductive, copulatory—the human penis is unique among primates in the absence of a penile bone, which could be easily fractured and incapacitated as he stands upright and walks on two legs.

THE HOT ZONE

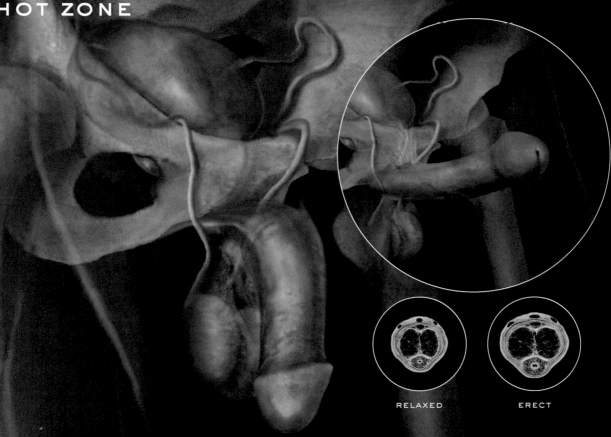

RELAXED   ERECT

SAME BEGINNING, DIFFERENT ENDINGS

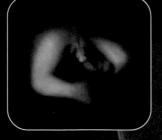

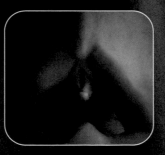

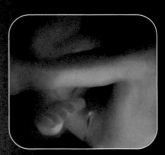

7TH WEEK MALE OR FEMALE   3RD-MONTH MALE   3RD-MONTH FEMALE

In part, hydraulic action also accounts for female sexual pleasure. Blood fills the capillary net in the vaginal walls, literally squeezing moisture out of the cells around it; with no place else to go, mucus seeps into the vagina, which like the penis is engineered for more than one function (it also plays a role in reproduction). The clitoris, on the other hand, has one purpose only—excitation—the product of extraordinary bioelectrics.

Pea-sized, it contains a charged hive of 8,000 nerve endings, twice as many as the much larger penis and the most of any external structure in the body including fingers, lips, and tongue. Freud disastrously underestimated the clitoris as "the only bodily organ which is really regarded as inferior": "the atrophied penis," he called it. In fact, as Angier writes, in terms of sensation, "a woman's little brain is bigger than a man's."

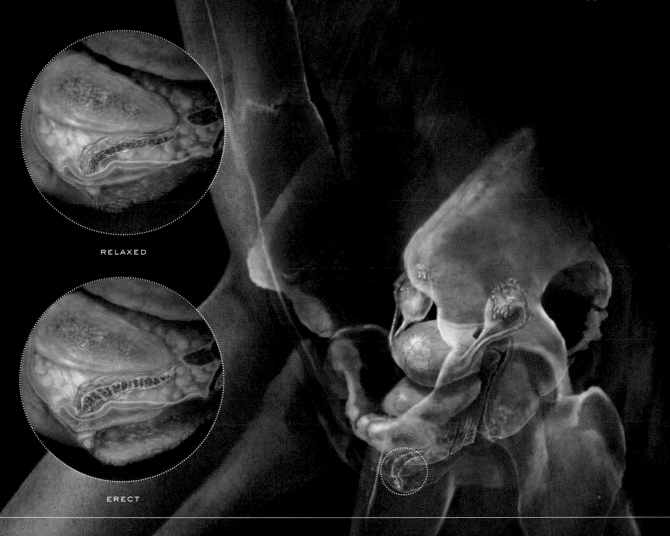

RELAXED

ERECT

In both biological and design terms, the development of the sex organs starts with indifference; that is, males and females are the same. Though genetically already assigned, the gender of a 6-week-old embryo is physiologically indistinguishable, even as primitive sex cords, 2 thick ridges of sexually determined cells, first arise. Approaching the end of the second month, the internal sex organs, including ovaries and testicles, develop. Not until the third month do the vagina and penis start to form, and when they do, the initial protrusion is shaped and molded in such a way that it can produce characteristics familiar to both. This Rorschach-like structure is called the *indifferent penis*, which makes it sound like another name for a 25-year-old slacker who's just split up with his lover.

DESIGNED TO FIT

The second-century Greek physician Galen observed of the snug complementarity between the male and female genitals, "Turn outward the woman's, turn inward, so to speak, and fold double the man's, and you will find both the same in every respect." Mirror-image homology, however, is just the physical set-up. The biomechanics of mating are kickstarted by arousal.

As we become sexually excited, our sex organs prepare for coitus through changes in the circulatory and nervous systems. The brain, receiving signals from the genitals, is tantalized, anticipating erotic pleasure. Our hearts hasten, flooding our arteries, while our veins constrict. Blood engorges the erectile tissue of the penis and clitoris as well as the testicles, ovaries, and labia minora—two thin folds of integument that lie just inside the vestibule of the vagina. Muscles tense. Nipples stiffen.

These effects plateau. In a woman, the outer third of the vagina becomes vasoconstricted, moistening, while the inner two thirds expand slightly and the uterus becomes elevated—all in preparation for receiving sperm. Male pre-ejaculate adds lubrication near the cervix. Not our exertions but our involuntary nervous systems increase breathing and quicken pulses.

Orgasm occurs with a loss of control, a shuddering release something like a sneeze. In men, this occurs in two stages. As the intensity builds, reflex centers in the spinal cord send impulses to the genitals, prompting the smooth muscles of the testes, epididymides, and vasa deferentia to contract and squeeze sperm into the urethra. It's the filling of the urethra that triggers the muscles encasing the base of the penis to contract and force the semen out. Women's orgasms involve the uterus, outer vagina, and clitoris but not the inner regions of the vagina. Typically harder to stimulate than men, yet capable, once excited, of multiple orgasms, women appreciate gentle, sustained stimulation.

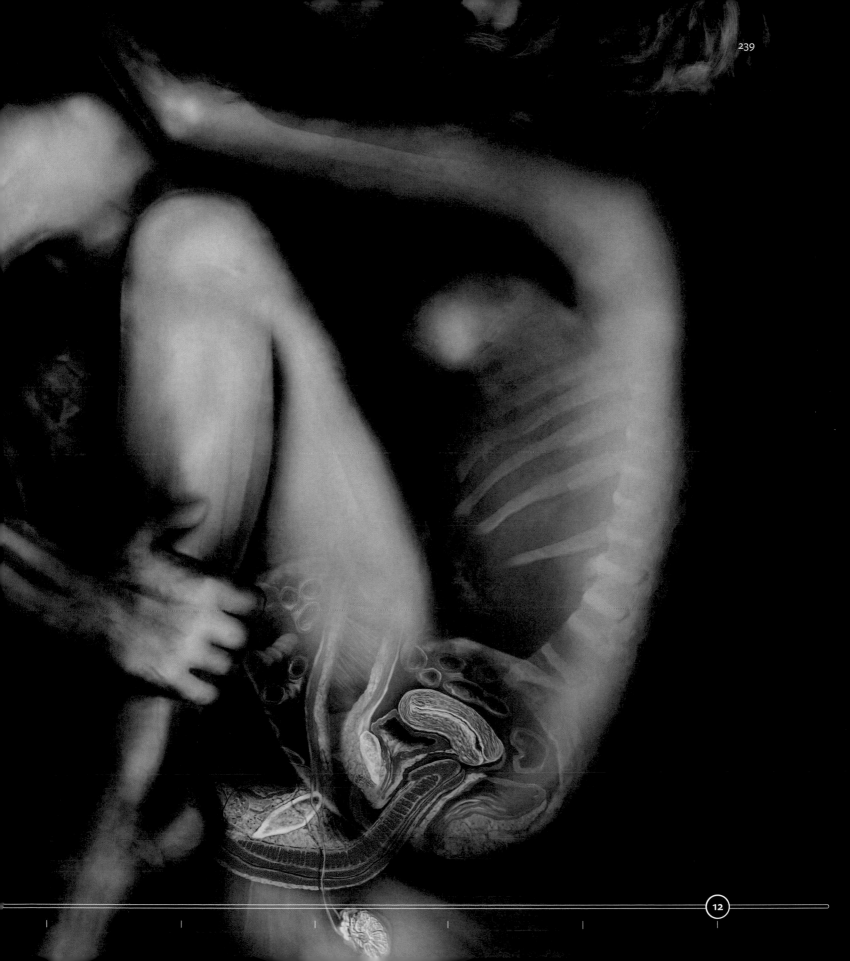

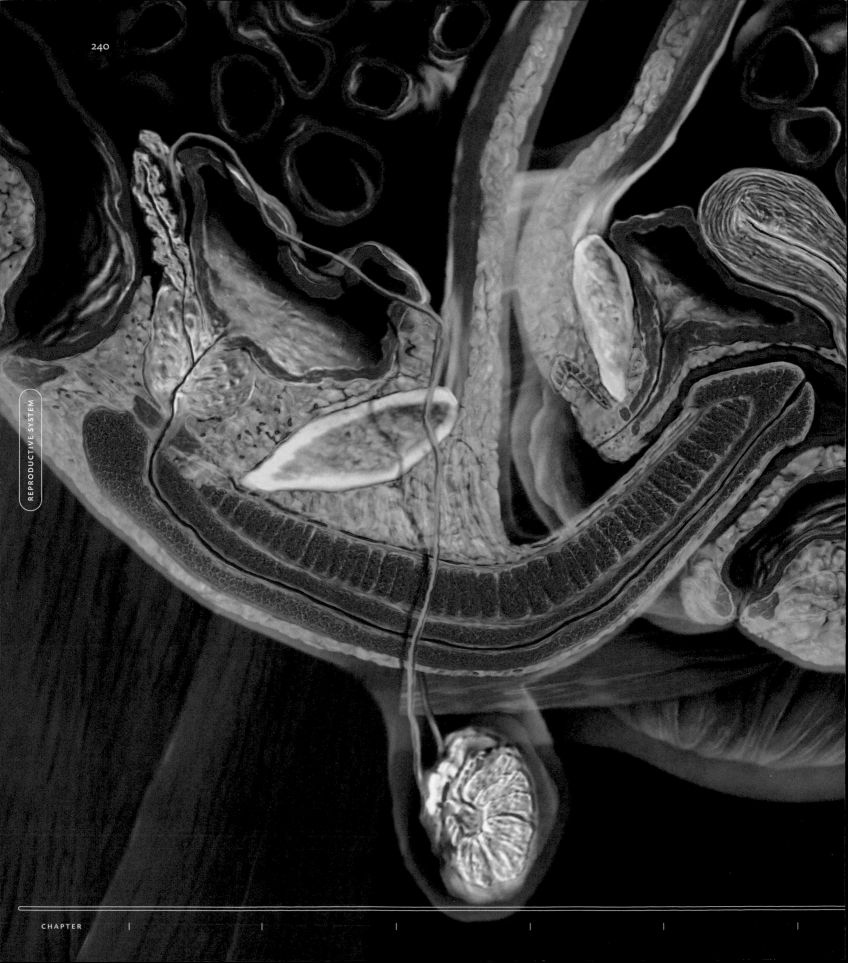

UPON ORGASM, THE UTERUS AND CERVIX REPEATEDLY DIP DOWN AND UP LIKE A PLUNGER DRAWING THE SPERM UPWARD INTO THE UTERUS. RECENT RESEARCH HAS LEAD TO A NEW THEORY WHICH HYPOTHESIZES THAT IT IS THESE DENSE, MUSCULAR CONTRACTIONS OF THE UTERUS THAT ARE RESPONSIBLE FOR THE ACCELERATION OF THE SPERM TOWARD THE EGG, AND NOT THE FLAGELLUM OF THE SPERM, AS HAS BEEN THE CONVENTIONAL BELIEF.

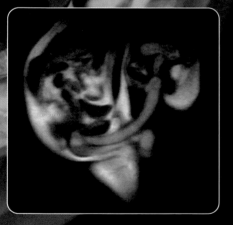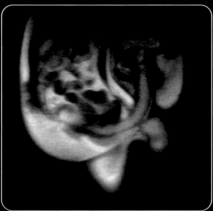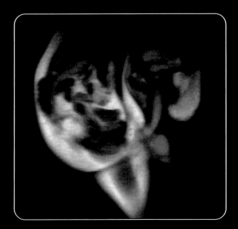

FACE TO FACE

With the exception of one species of monkey, humans are the only animals who can mate while looking at each others' faces. As part of the "bipedal" family of mammals, the sex organs of the male and female are not oriented from the back as is the case for most mammals who naturally mate with the male approaching from behind the female. The female's downward-tipping vagina extends toward the back of her body internally and suggests that copulation face to face is natural and most suitable. With modern technology, such as Magnetic Resonance Imaging (MRI), the internal character-istics of the male and female anatomies can be seen during intercourse (ABOVE).

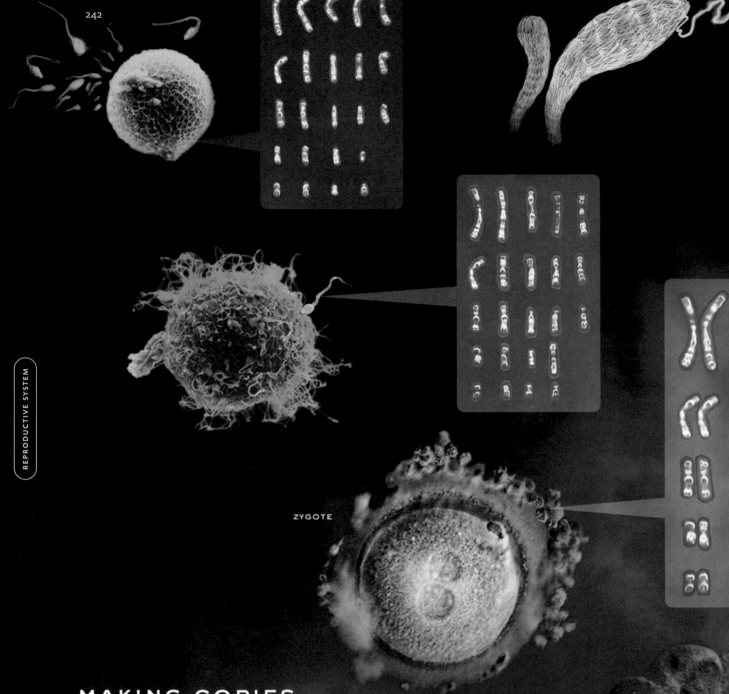

ZYGOTE

MAKING COPIES
(FERTILIZATION)

Once a sperm penetrates the ovum, their nuclei fuse and a single new cell (zygote) is produced that contains genetic instructions from both parents. The information is encoded on genes, strung like pop beads along 23 pairs of linear threads (chromosomes) in the nucleus. Each gene synthesizes a copy of itself from available chemicals. Then the chromosomes split lengthwise, minting 2 half-chromosomes, each of which promptly moves aside so that when the cell itself pancakes and splits, as if being pulled by a drawstring into equal halves, each with its own nucleus, its DNA is a perfect copy, intact and ready to repeat the process.

The origami of cells dividing and differentiating into new forms begins indolently. After waiting almost 2 days to cleave

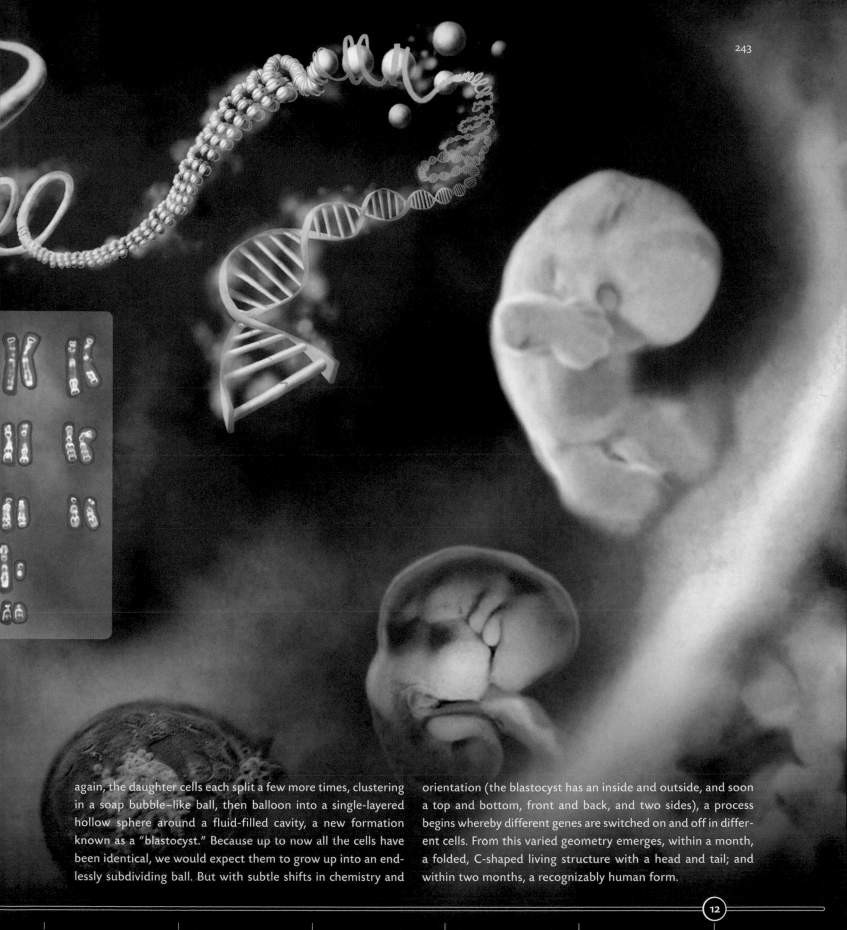

again, the daughter cells each split a few more times, clustering in a soap bubble–like ball, then balloon into a single-layered hollow sphere around a fluid-filled cavity, a new formation known as a "blastocyst." Because up to now all the cells have been identical, we would expect them to grow up into an end-lessly subdividing ball. But with subtle shifts in chemistry and orientation (the blastocyst has an inside and outside, and soon a top and bottom, front and back, and two sides), a process begins whereby different genes are switched on and off in differ-ent cells. From this varied geometry emerges, within a month, a folded, C-shaped living structure with a head and tail; and within two months, a recognizably human form.

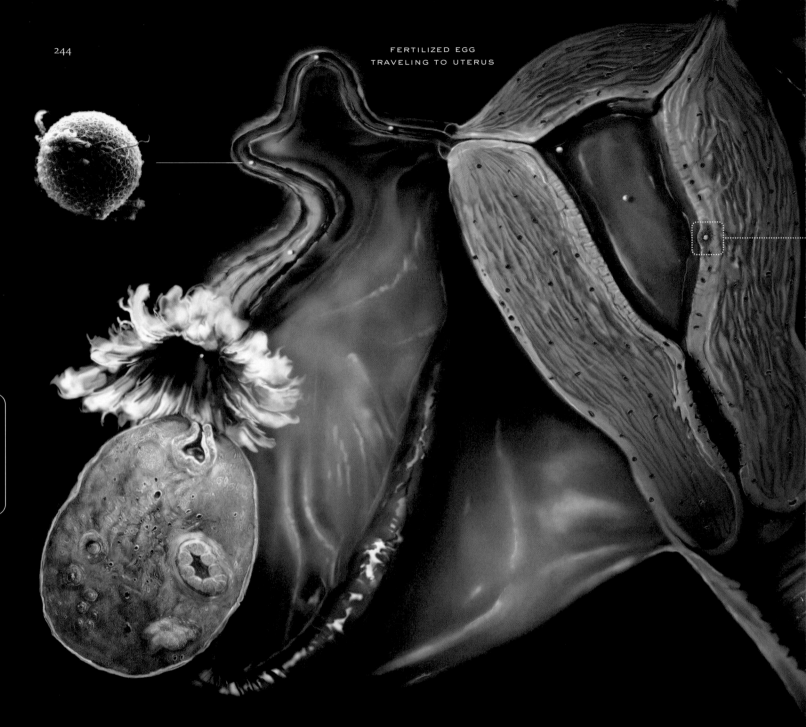

NESTLING

· After fertilization, the second great challenge of reproduction is the joining of 2 lives—embryo and mother. The
blastocyst, a parasitic, barely visible dot measuring less than
$^1/_{100}$ of an inch across, is swept along the length of the
fallopian tube and tumbles into the uterus. Meanwhile,
hormones from the abandoned follicles in the mother's
ovaries bathe the uterine lining, making it soft, porous, and
absorbent—receptive. As cells along the rim of the blastocyst secreting machetelike enzymes to erode the uterine
lining, make contact, they latch on. Rupturing the mother's
capillaries, these rim cells fuse into a tough protective
membrane (chorion). Burrowing farther, the blastocyst
becomes awash in the mother's starch-rich blood, and
fingerlike structures from inside the chorion reach out and

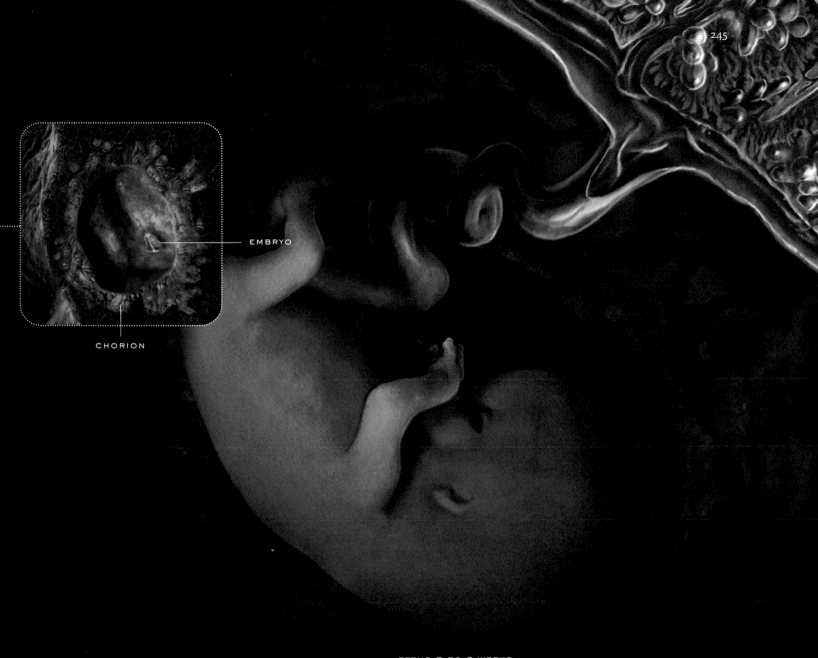

EMBRYO

CHORION

FETUS 7 TO 8 WEEKS

tap the mother's circulation. (Vampire myths may originate in the unconscious recollection of this earliest mother-child encounter.) The ideal site for implantation is located on the back wall of the uterus, near the support and protection of the spine.

A disk-shaped mass of blood-rich tissues soon emerges from the blastula to form an exchange organ (placenta) between the chorion and the uterine wall. Blood vessels from the mother and embryo intertwine in the placenta without actually joining, allowing stale blood to be exchanged for fresh, waste products for nourishment, embryonic hormones for maternal hormones, all while barring the passage of infection and most other harmful agents.

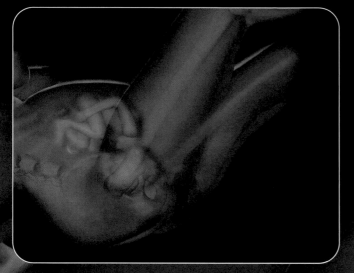
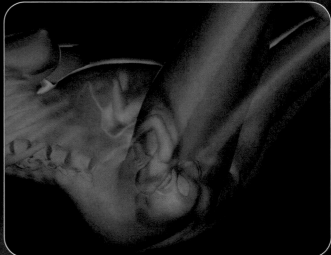

EXPULSION (GREETING A NEW WORLD)

Biomechanically, a woman's reproductive system becomes, at birth, a kind of pump, as the same organs that once coordinated sexual maturation, delicately handled the transfer of male DNA during conception, then for 9 months served as an incubator, combine to expel a writhing baby that has gotten too big.

Gentle uterine contractions at the onset of labor prompt a positive feedback loop with the pituitary, which secretes oxytocin, the so-called "love hormone," inducing even stronger contractions. Another hormone secreted by the ovaries relaxes the cervix, the sphincter at the base of the uterus that, stretched by the baby's head, prepares to widen gradually from a half-centimeter—about the size of a peanut—to 10 centimeters in diameter. Meanwhile the vagina, relaxing and stretching to allow passage, secretes a complex carbohydrate called glycogen, which metabolizes on the spot to lactic acid, an infection-fighting agent.

When the contractions, which are involuntary, come every 2 to 3 minutes and last about a minute, a woman can safely bear down and push hard with her abdominal muscles.

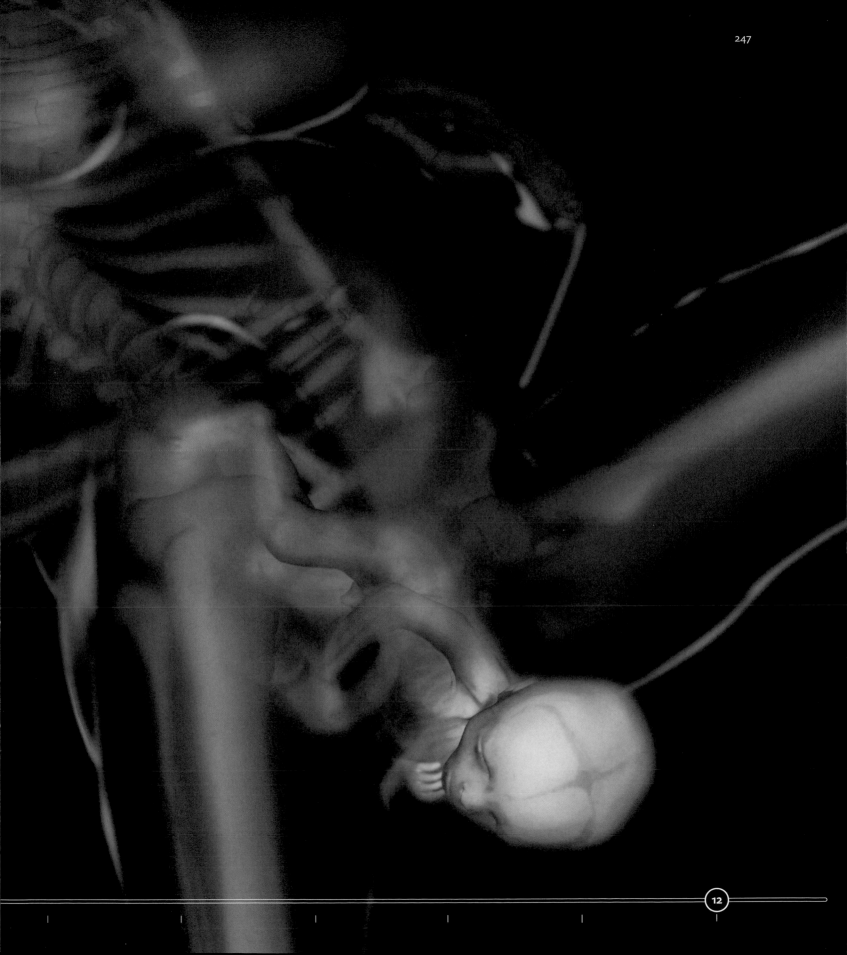

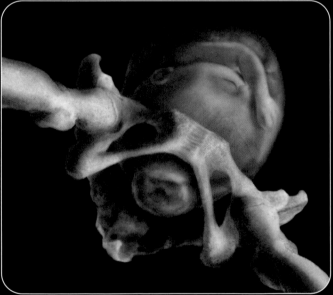

BEFORE, DURING, AND AFTER PREGNANCY

THE UTERUS: During pregnancy, the uterus expands to hold up to 1,000 times its normal capacity and gains weight due to an increase in muscle fiber. Afterward, hormones work to restore it to its original size and shape.

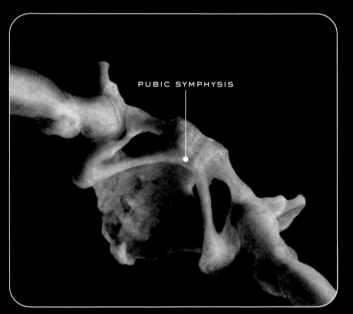

PUBIC SYMPHYSIS

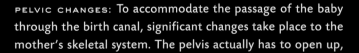

PELVIC CHANGES: To accommodate the passage of the baby through the birth canal, significant changes take place to the mother's skeletal system. The pelvis actually has to open up, like a hinge, from the back, which results in the stretching, and sometimes tearing, of the ligaments and cartilage that joins the pelvis anteriorly (in the front).

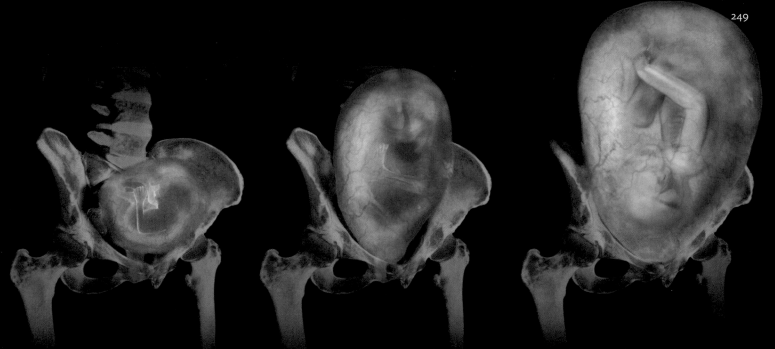

BREASTS BEFORE AND AFTER: Mammary glands double in size in anticipation of breast feeding, and the small glands around the nipple may become raised and lumpy and change color. Breasts resist returning to their original state as the mammary glands shrink, mainly because the connective tissue between them has become overly stretched.

BEFORE PREGNANCY   LACTATING   AFTER NURSING

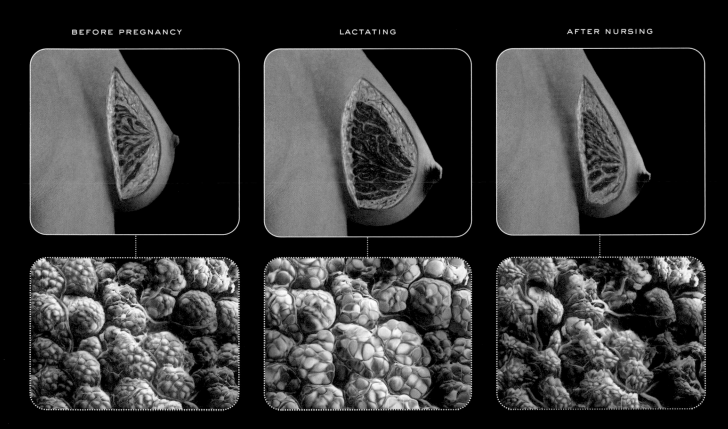

MIRRORED IN NATURE

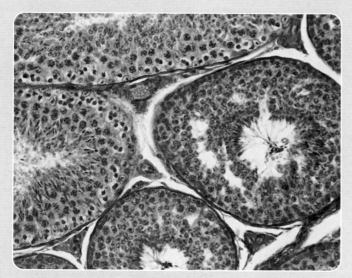

SEMINIFEROUS TUBULES WHERE SPERM DEVELOP

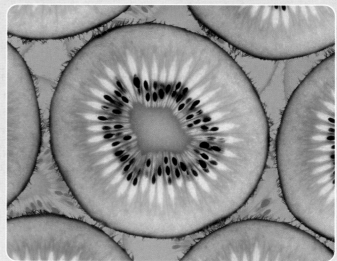

KIWI FRUIT SLICES WITH DEVELOPING SEEDS

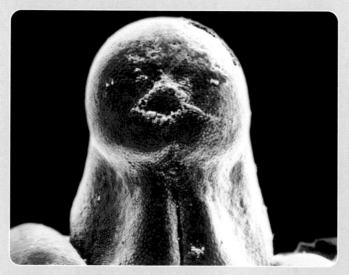

EXTERNAL GENITALIA IN EMBRYO

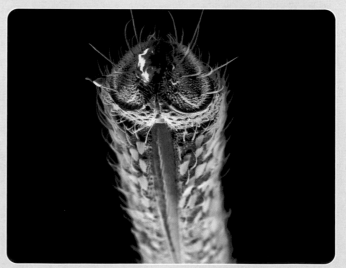

MOSQUITO PROBOSCIS

It is as a mechanism, or a mechanical construction,
that the physicist looks upon the world.
—D'Arcy Thompson

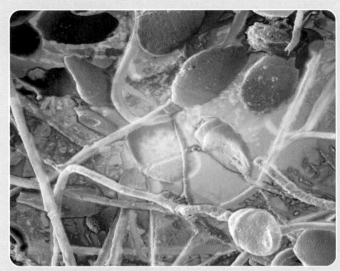

THE MALE SEX CELL, SPERM

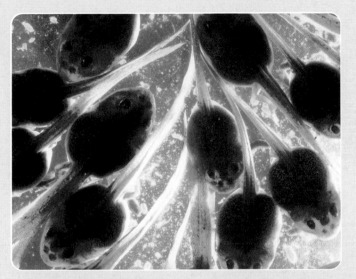

METAMORPHOSING TADPOLES

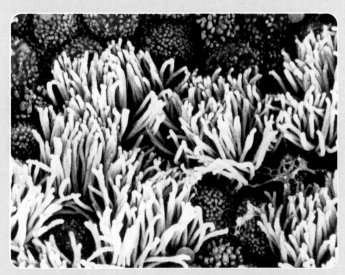

INTERIOR SURFACE OF THE FALLOPIAN TUBE, CILIA, AND MICROVILLI

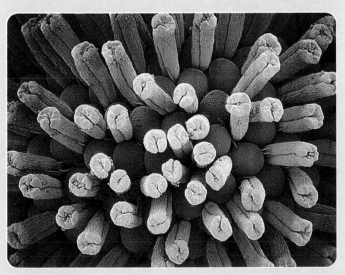

FLOWER PISTILS

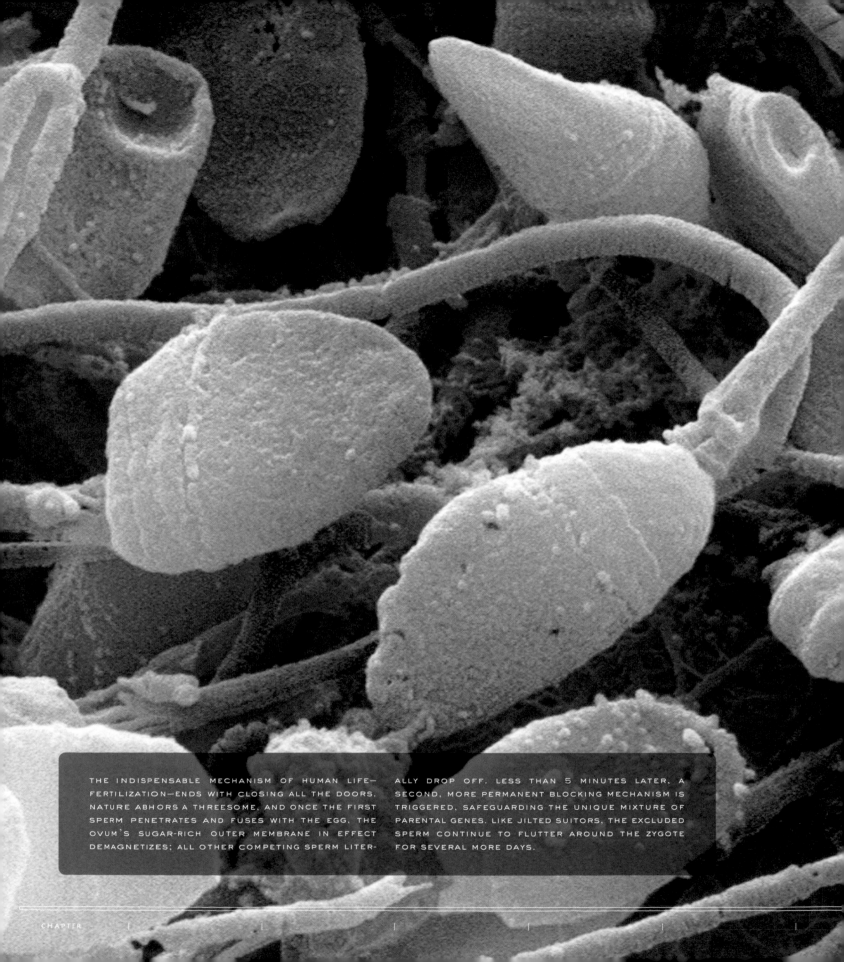

THE INDISPENSABLE MECHANISM OF HUMAN LIFE— FERTILIZATION—ENDS WITH CLOSING ALL THE DOORS. NATURE ABHORS A THREESOME, AND ONCE THE FIRST SPERM PENETRATES AND FUSES WITH THE EGG, THE OVUM'S SUGAR-RICH OUTER MEMBRANE IN EFFECT DEMAGNETIZES; ALL OTHER COMPETING SPERM LITER- ALLY DROP OFF. LESS THAN 5 MINUTES LATER, A SECOND, MORE PERMANENT BLOCKING MECHANISM IS TRIGGERED, SAFEGUARDING THE UNIQUE MIXTURE OF PARENTAL GENES. LIKE JILTED SUITORS, THE EXCLUDED SPERM CONTINUE TO FLUTTER AROUND THE ZYGOTE FOR SEVERAL MORE DAYS.

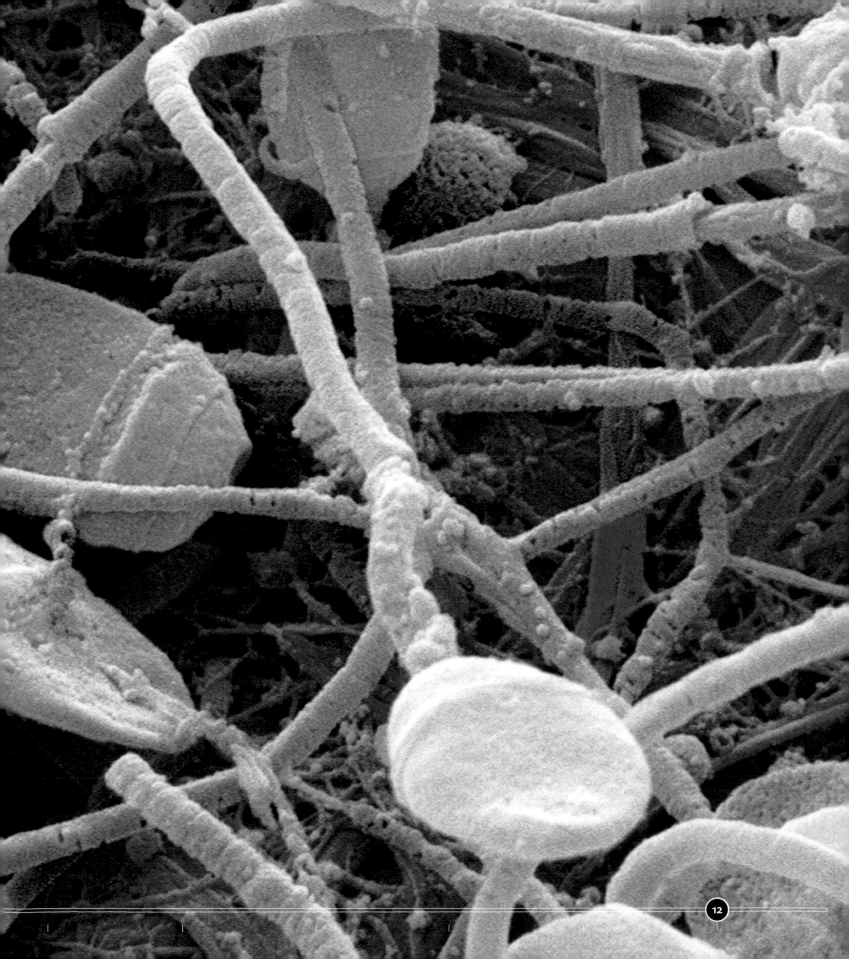

ACKNOWLEDGMENTS

My family: Susan and Andreas
For supporting me emotionally, professionally, and spiritually, even through the times I had doubts, and most importantly for helping me to feel and understand a unique love that I treasure each morning I wake and see you both.

Bill Thomas, Editor in Chief, Doubleday Books
I want to thank Bill for his continued faith in our work. He succeeds in continuing to make my publishing with Doubleday among the most fulfilling professional experiences of my career.

Kendra Harpster, Associate Editor, Doubleday Books
Many thanks for her devotion to our work and this book. As well as being a pleasure to work with, her patience, capacity for problem solving, and her editorial style have helped tremendously to improve the vision of this book.

Adrianne Noe, Director of the
National Museum of Health and Medicine of the Armed Forces Institute of Pathology.
I want to thank Adrianne for her very smart and warm encouragement of our work. I truly treasure our intellectual exchange and friendship.

Eric Baker Design Associates, Inc.:
Eric Baker and Cindy Goldstein
For their creative design and ease of collaboration

Barry Werth: writer
For yet another Mozartian text

Anatomical Travelogue participants:
Ann Canapary, Attila Ambrus, Attila Zalanyi, Benjamin Lipman, Betty Lee, Casey Steffen, Chad Capeland, Donghyun Han, Elias Papatheodorou, Glenn Ball, Ildiko McGivney, Jean-Claude Michel, Jeremy Mack, Karina Metcalf, Laszlo Balogh, Levente Szileszky, Mark Mallari, Matt Wimsatt, Poy Yee, Taryn McLaughlin

E. C. Lockett, Imaging Specialist
National Museum of Health and Medicine of the Armed Forces Institute of Pathology

Center for In Vivo Microscopy
Department of Radiology
Duke University Medical Center

Biomedical Magnetic Resonance Laboratory
University of Illinois, College of Medicine at Urbana-Champaign

Marlin Minks
Photography, Anatomical Travelogue

P. Schwartz and H. W. Michelmann
University of Göettingen, Germany

The National Institute of Child Health and Human
Development (NICHHD) National Institute of Health

Douglas T. Carrell, Ph.D., H.C.L.D.
Associate Professor of Surgery, Obstetrics
and Gynecology, and Physiology,
Director of IVF and Andrology Laboratories
and
Benjamin R. Emery, B.S.
University of Utah School of Medicine

Lewis C. Krey Ph.D., Anna Blaszczyk M.S.,
Caroline McCaffrey Ph.D. and Alexis Adler B.S.
Program for In Vitro Fertilization,
Reproductive Surgery and Infertility
Department of Obstetrics and Gynecology
New York University School of Medicine

E. Scott Pretorius, MD
Associate Chair, Education, Department of Radiology
Assistant Professor
University of Pennsylvania Health Systems

Professor Katerina Harvati
Assistant Professor of Physical Anthropology
New York University

Professor Todd Olson
Director of Clinical Anatomy
Albert Einstein College of Medicine

Sebastian Tille and Buddy Bossmann
Carl Zeiss MicroImaging, Inc.

Doug Morris, Ph.D.
Staff Scientist
National Institutes of Health
National Institute of Neurological Disease and Stroke
NIH Magnetic Resonance Facility

Professor Steven Frost
Assistant Professor of Physical Anthropology
University of Oregon

Hoby Hetherington, Ph.D.
Albert Einstein College of Medicine
Department of Radiology

New York University Medical Center
Department of Radiology

Donald Lindberg, MD

The National Library of Medicine (NLM)

National Institutes of Health

Kim Cacho
Doubleday Production

Bob Levin
Levine Plotkin & Menin, LLP

Thanks to Michael Rosenstein of AMD

Images were produced on systems using
AMD Opteron™ processors

Scientific visualization and volumes software developed in collaboration with Volume Graphics GmbH, Germany (www.volumegraphics.com). We would also like to thank Christof, Christoph, Thomas, and the team at Volume Graphics for their extraordinary work and support.

All stock imagery is from the Science Source division of Photo Researchers Inc. www.sciencesource.com

Special Thanks to:
Tomas Dankos
Kristen Patrick
Pillar Regan
Timea Resan
Christina Wood